D0192081

You Can Fight for Your Life

Lawrence LeShan

YOU CAN FIGHT FOR YOUR LIFE

Emotional Factors in the Treatment of Cancer

M. EVANS AND COMPANY, INC.
New York, New York 10017

LIBRARY OF CONGRESS CATALOGING IN PUBLICATION DATA

LeShan, Lawrence L   1920-
    You can fight for your life: emotional factors
in the causation of cancer.

        1. Cancer—Psychological aspects.   2. Carcino-
genesis—Psychological aspects.   I. Title.
RC263.L37   616.9′94′08   76-30464
ISBN 0-87131-234-4 (casebound)
ISBN 0-87131-494-0 (paperback)

M. Evans and Company, Inc.
216 East 49th Street
New York, New York 10017

Design by Joel Schick

Manufactured in the United States of America

19 18 17 16 15 14 13 12 11 10

There are a hundred names, and more—
the brave companions, the pioneers, who
trusted me and helped me learn; who
struggled with courage and passion beyond
describing to search out the roots of their
pathology—to reach for what they had
never dared to reach before: the wonder
and beauty of being themselves. "I know I
won't make it," some said, "but maybe
someone else will, from what we learned
together." How I wish I could tell them
that was true.

LAWRENCE LESHAN
October, 1976

Contents

	Foreword	*ix*
	Introduction	*xi*
	Appreciation	*xvii*
1	The First Clues	*1*
2	The Search for a Pattern	*14*
3	A Fuller Picture Emerges	*28*
4	The Emotional Life History of Cancer Patients	*49*
5	Stress and Susceptibility	*73*
6	Psychotherapy and the Cancer Patient	*95*
7	I Want to Live	*115*
8	The Third Road	*131*
9	The World of the Cancer Patient	*162*
10	What It Means to Fight for One's Life	*179*
	Selected Bibliography	*187*

Foreword

This book, *You Can Fight for Your Life,* represents the work of one of the most courageous men of our times. The research that is presented here is some of the most important that has been done in medicine. To have undertaken the formidable task of solidifying the link between the emotions and cancer at the time Dr. LeShan began his study is more than is reasonable to ask of any human. That he accomplished it in ten years is something for which we can be forever grateful. His background and methods as an experimental psychologist and his skill as a clinician were joined in the writing of this book to make the necessary steps in logic that clarify the elusive relationship between the mind and cancer.

It is important to remember the very great love and personal sacrifice that has gone into the work that this book represents: the great difficulty of gaining patient access for a non-physician, the ridicule suffered at the hands of those who could not see his vision, the intense emotional pain that comes when exploring with patients why they live and why they die, the extreme loss that comes from loving patients—being deeply involved with them and then standing by impotently as they die in their struggle. The great emotional price this extracted from Dr. LeShan as he proceeded was paid by sacrificing aspects of himself, his family, his life. It is impossible to appreciate fully the great strength and courage of Dr. LeShan as reflected in this book. Unless one has walked some of this road, there is no adequate frame of reference to realize the amount of pain experienced while receiving professional criticism and observing family pain, with the only reward being personal satisfaction.

This book is of great help to the professional—doctor, nurse, counselor, member of the clergy—and most of all to the patient and family in understanding this most elusive connection between the emotions and cancer.

O. Carl Simonton, M.D.

Introduction

The fact of anxiety in everyday life is of no less concern to the medical profession than the infectious diseases of a generation or two ago. The 1979 report of the United States Surgeon General points out that in 1900 four diseases—tuberculosis, diphtheria, poliomyelitis, and gastroenteritis—were high on the list of killers. Those same four diseases, however, produced a combined total of only 10,000 deaths in 1978. If the incidence of those diseases were the same in 1978 as it had been in 1900, the death toll would have exceeded 875,000.

Based on such developments, and on the increase in

longevity to the mid-seventies for the average person, the Surgeon General's report concludes that the American people are healthier than ever before. But that same report also calls attention to the prevalence of anxiety as a major health threat and to the problems represented by the widespread use of drugs, especially in the category of tranquilizers.

Can anxiety lead to serious disease? Many medical investigators contend that there is hardly a major illness that cannot be triggered by profound anxiety. Even cancer can have its origins in emotional tensions or disturbances. Depression and despair make their registrations not just in the mind but in the body. Contemporary medical researchers have been able to make correlations between emotional disturbances and malignancies. For the past quarter of a century, the psychiatric literature has carried studies by such names as Bahnson, Kissen, LeShan, Reznikoff, Schmale, and Iker. They have been probing non-physiological causes of some cancers and have attempted to identify the personality types in which prolonged despair, depression, or other emotional disturbances tend to escalate into malignances. Lawrence LeShan is prominent among those who have attempted to deal with cancer preventively by helping to educate cancer-prone personalities to make essential adjustments in their attitudes to stress and in their ability to cope with situations that might otherwise lead to dangerous anxiety and depression.

While many of these approaches are relatively new, it should be emphasized that the connection between malignancies and the emotions was recognized at least eighteen hundred years ago. Galen, who was born in the second century A.D. and was the most eminent physician-philosopher of his time, observed that women who suffered from melancholy had a greater tendency to develop breast cancers than did women of more positive disposition and outlook. Similar observations have been made over the course of the centuries, especially in the past two hundred years. But it is only recently that the more particularized approaches to an understanding of the connection between cancer and the emotions have been systematically pursued.

One especially compelling line of research, discussed in this book, concerns the ability of the individual to exercise some degree of control over his or her autonomic nervous system and thus contribute effectively to the battle against serious disease. The notion is widespread that inner workings of the human system—circulation of the blood, reproduction of cells, endocrine system, heart functions, and so on—are completely beyond the reach of the conscious intelligence. It is of course true that these functions occur without our being aware of them. But this fact does not mean that they are entirely beyond our control. Some of the most dramatic medical research in recent years has been in the field of self-control. At the Menninger Foundation headquarters in Topeka, Kansas, for example, patients are taught in the biofeedback laboratory to relieve migraine headaches and high blood pressure. They learn how to increase the flow of blood to the hands at will. This particular exercise is a potent factor in relieving migraine and in reducing blood pressure. Some 350 cases have been documented in support of this approach.

Not all human illnesses, of course, are treatable through self-control techniques, but medical intervention works much better when the resources of the patient are fully engaged. These resources are not mythical. The human body possesses a highly developed healing system which in the overwhelming majority of cases is adequate to its challenges. In cases where the balance of forces is negative, help may be needed. Even in such severe instances, however, it is known that the healing system can be depressed or enhanced depending on the emotional environment. The panic and uncertainty that are the almost inevitable products of serious disease can actually intensify the underlying condition, thus setting the stage for a chain reaction in which the mood deepens the illness and the illness the mood. That is why the physician must be a humane psychologist and not just a trained scientist. He knows that his medications and his other ministrations can be much more effective when the patient's panic is crowded out by the will to live, buoyant hopes, confidence in the physician and in oneself.

Is there any scientific basis for the belief that the positive emotions have specific physiological effects? It has long been known that the negative emotions cause specific downside chemical effects on the body, but it is only recently that medical researchers have begun to accumulate evidence that the positive emotions also produce chemical changes. The picture now emerging is of the brain not just as the seat of consciousness but as a gland—the most prolific gland in the human body. Year by year, the number of secretions produced by the brain that have been identified has increased steadily.

Some neurologists have stated that the number is at least 380—and they are confident that during the next decade brain researchers may identify twice or three times that number. What is now definitely known is that the brain produces a vast array of encephalins and endorphins—morphine-like substances that not only counteract pain but help to set a stage for recovery. The brain also has a role in the production of gamma globulin, the vital substance of the immunological system. Recently developed knowledge about the brain has called public attention to the production of interferon, a cancer-blocking substance.

Since all these secretions are directly involved in the maintenance of health and in overcoming disease, it is natural to wonder whether the conscious intelligence has any part to play in their functioning or whether they exist completely apart from the emotional and intellectual forces and climate. One thing appears likely: under circumstances of depression, despair, panic, fear, exasperation, and frustration, the healing resources of the human brain are not fully engaged. Under circumstances of a robust will to live and great expectations, however, the ability of the brain to generate chemical change is enhanced.

Such at least is the evidence that is now emerging

You Can Fight for Your Life

from brain research being done at centers like Stanford University, Harvard University, the University of California at San Francisco, the University of California at Los Angeles, Southern Illinois University, and at least a dozen other research centers in this country and elsewhere. Lawrence LeShan uses this fast-developing knowledge in helping individuals to understand their ability to get the most out of their healing capacities and to adopt a design for living that can promote good health.

Norman Cousins

Appreciation

First and foremost, I must thank Richard E. Worthington, Ph.D., for sharing with me his first thoughts about a relationship between cancer and personality—and for the faith he showed in my ability to research this question by providing the first grant for this work. The project would have been short-lived, however, if Frederick Ayer, II, through the Ayer Foundation, had not shown an interest, an enthusiasm, a guidance and a determination to see it through, far beyond the kind of support research workers dare to hope for. It is almost unheard of in the area of scientific research for a foundation to support a project long enough for the researcher himself to feel he has finished his task!

After I had obtained these research funds, I found, much to my surprise, that no hospital, no research center in the entire metropolitan area of New York would permit me to set foot in their establishment, although at that time all I required were cancer patients to interview and test (if the patients wished to do so). In some cases medical directors and other hospital personnel told me privately they suspected I might be on an important quest but I would give their institution "a bad name." One research group, the Institute of Applied Biology, dared to permit my investigations. The Director, Emmanuel Revici, M.D., said to me, "We know there must be some intervening variables we don't understand, because it is almost impossible to predict, in medical terms, who will recover from cancer and who will die. Perhaps you are on the right track—only time will tell. I have no way of knowing if you are a charlatan or not, at this point; time will tell. *But you have a right to explore.*"

In the course of the research, which eventually extended to working on an international level, there were a few individuals who were especially instrumental in making me think hard and critically about what I was doing. To mention four of the most meaningful relationships with colleagues: David Kissen, M.D., Gotthard Booth, M.D., Graham Bennette, M.D., and Edgar N. Jackson, most of all.

Because of the nature of my work—dealing almost

constantly with terminally ill patients—I was in a constant state of mourning and grief, as so many people whom I had come to care about so much died. It would have been impossible to function effectively, much less survive as a human being, without extraordinary support. The control therapist, who believed in my work—and in me—and who was always ready with wise insights, affection and constant encouragement was Marthe Gassmann, M.D.

There were two constant companions to my adventure, and now, looking back over the years, I wonder and marvel at the loving approval, support and encouragement they gave me. One was my daughter Wendy, who as a little girl somehow managed to feel more proud than rejected by the inevitable preoccupation of my work, and the other was my wife, Eda, who was, ultimately, the partner who made it all possible.

I owe this book to the interest and encouragement of Herbert Katz, and to the understanding and enthusiasm (and writing skills) of John Malone.

Lawrence LeShan

You Can Fight for Your Life

The First Clues 1

Cancer is not just one disease. It is a variety of related diseases that affect different parts of the human body in a diverse number of ways. And, partially for this reason, it remains the most mysterious of all major diseases. Over the past several decades, fortunately, a great deal of progress has been made in dealing with cancer from a strictly medical point of view: new surgical procedures have been perfected, chemotherapy and radiation treatments have proved effective in many cases, and further experiments ranging from the use of new drugs to the application of high temperatures to

1

affected parts of the body hold out the promise of additional help for the cancer victim. Yet the mysteries remain. Despite all the advances in treatment, the *causes* of cancer remain a subject of speculation and controversy.

After two decades of work with cancer patients, however, I believe that I can offer some new evidence and some fresh insights into the reasons why some individuals get cancer while others do not, and into the factors that make it possible for some cancer victims to fight successfully for their lives while others rapidly succumb to the disease. I am a psychotherapist and not a medical researcher. But, on the basis of my work with dozens of terminal cancer patients in intensive psychotherapy, as well as extensive study of the personality of hundreds of other cancer victims, there is a generalization that I believe can be made with great certainty: the presence of cancer is usually an indication that there is something else wrong in the life of the patient. The cancer victim usually has a psychological orientation that increases the chances of getting cancer and makes it more difficult for many individuals to fight for their lives when they do develop a malignancy.

Nearly all the cancer patients who have come to me for psychotherapy have been terminal patients. In almost all cases, their life expectancy was minimal. They continued, of course, under medical treatment. It was the job of their physicians, chemotherapists, and nurses to alleviate the patients' pain and to attempt to slow the spread of their cancers by medical means. It has been my job to try to help these patients, through psychotherapy, to develop or regain their will to live. It has been my job to locate that "something else" that was wrong, to uncover the roots of that psychological orientation that prevents many cancer patients from using their human resources to fight the disease, that "something else" that I have come to believe is linked to the development of the disease in the first place. A number of my patients are still alive today, many years after their cases were diagnosed as medically hopeless.

My work in the cancer field has not involved the study of cells under a microscope. I have worked with people—individuals. There have been 71 of them. Each was unique, yet all were linked by a number of common threads. This is their story more than it is mine. What they have to tell us about despair, and about learning to hope, goes beyond the mysteries of cancer itself. Their story is about what it means to be alive.

I remember Jenny.

Like all my other patients, when I first met her Jenny was dying of cancer. Her malignancy had spread too far and too fast for an operation to be of any use. In her quiet voice, Jenny told me that she was not surprised at this outcome to her life. She had always felt that nothing would ever go right for her, that she had no real hope of happiness. For some years before the cancer struck, she had undergone traditional psychotherapy in an attempt to discover what it was that prevented her from developing any sense of fulfillment, or achieving any hope for the future. The answer had continued to elude her, however, and when she got cancer she saw it as just one more example of the fruitlessness of her life.

After her illness was diagnosed, and it was determined that she was beyond medical help, she came to me for therapy. At that time I was working with a number of cancer patients, in a program at the Institute of Applied Biology. I was trying to develop new methods for dealing with the particular problems of cancer patients, and at the same time carrying forward a research project concerning the possible connection between personality and the incidence of cancer.

Jenny had been coming to me for several months when she said something to me one day that summed up precisely what my work with cancer patients was all about. "You know," she said with a slight smile, "this is a strange kind of psychotherapy. You go along and it's very pleasant and interesting, and you are learning a lot and there's no tension about it, and all of a sudden you find you're fighting for your life." She paused, thought a moment, laughed, and added, "I guess I meant that last phrase, 'fighting for your life,' in both senses."

Jenny could not have said anything more encouraging to me than those words. They indicated that she had indeed begun to have some hope for herself as a person, regardless of how long she had to live. And they indicated that she had come to believe, as I did, that one *could* fight for one's life, that the cancer in her body did not exist independently of the way she felt about her life, but was, in fact, related to it.

4

Cancer is a disease that raises innumerable questions —questions to which there sometimes seem to be almost as many answers, or partial answers, as there are people asking the questions. Currently, the main thrust of cancer research is in the area of environmental factors —a massive attempt to identify those substances in our world, whether natural or man-made, that may act as carcinogens. Such possible cancer-causing substances range from tobacco smoke to the synthetic estrogens found in certain drugs, from the asbestos in brake-linings and insulation to the vinyl-chloride widely used in the manufacture of plastics.

Such research is vital to our understanding of cancer-causing substances. But there are limitations to what laboratory research or statistics can tell us. There are continuing arguments among doctors and scientists as to whether a chemical that causes cancer in animals will do so in human beings. An additional problem lies in the fact that the latency period between exposure to a carcinogen and the development of an actual cancer can be as long as 35 years. Thus the development of cancer in young people, in their teens or twenties, is not adequately accounted for. But beyond these technical questions, a greater mystery remains. Why does one construction worker exposed to asbestos dust over a period of years develop cancer, while another man who has worked beside him does not? Why does one heavy smoker get lung cancer at forty, while another lives to be eighty with no problems?

A partial answer to these questions appears to lie in

5

genetics. Some people have an inherited predisposition, it seems, to the disease, just as others are prone to cataracts or hearing problems. But this answer only raises additional questions. To begin with, genetic research is one of the most complex fields of scientific endeavor—the number of variables to be considered is staggering. Any full explanation of why two of five siblings are struck by cancer while the other three are not seems to be a very long way off. And while genetics may partially explain why some people get cancer, it cannot encompass the fact that many cancer victims whose cases are regarded as hopeless continue to live for many years, and that in some cases their cancers undergo a remission, leaving the patients perfectly healthy once again. Take the case of John, for instance.

Twelve years ago, at the age of thirty-five, John began having severe headaches. A lawyer, John appeared to be leading a happy and successful life. He lived with his attractive wife and three children in a luxurious suburban home, and his position in his father's law firm assured a stable future.

Yet John was not living a life he would have chosen for himself. Although he had demonstrated unusual musical ability as a child, he had been timid and withdrawn. He found it difficult to communicate his true emotions and desires, and accepted the paths in life that his parents chose for him, becoming a lawyer to satisfy his father and even marrying the girl his mother picked out for him. Believing that he could win the love of others only by doing what they expected of him, he sacrificed his own dreams.

As a result, like Jenny, he felt trapped in an existence devoid of hope and empty of personal satisfaction. He hated working as a lawyer, and his marriage was marked by serious discord. Two years before his illness began, he had left his wife to attempt a career as a musician. But, unable to earn enough to support his family, and consumed by guilt, he returned home, giving up all hope of real happiness. A few months later, his headaches began.

An exploratory operation revealed a massive brain tumor, but the malignancy had developed to the point that nothing could be done except sew the incision back up again. He was told that he would not live for more than a few months. Paradoxically, the imminence of death seemed to release a new surge of inner strength. His doctors said that there was no known cure for a malignancy such as his, but instead of giving up, he searched for some unorthodox treatment that might help him. Reading about my work with a form of psychotherapy especially directed at terminal cancer patients—which was combined with the then new technique of chemotherapy—he decided to try this unusual approach and contacted us at the Institute of Applied Biology.

John remained at the institute for three years. In therapy with me he learned that it was possible to fight for his life. He began to work seriously on his music once again, and he divorced his wife. Today, John is in fine health, and is doing what he had always wanted for himself, working as a professional musician with a symphony orchestra.

Is John's cure a "miracle"? Or is it perhaps related to how he feels about himself and his world? As a man without hope, he developed cancer; as a man with new-found hope, his "terminal" cancer disappeared. Some of the processes by which John came to discover the hope in himself will be discussed in later chapters. For now, to put it simply, he came to understand that he could be loved for doing what he wanted with his life, and not just what others wanted for him. Once he became convinced of that, he was able to bring the full resources of his new-found sense of himself to the fight against the cancer within him. And he won that fight.

Clearly, the usual approaches to the problems of cancer do not adequately answer the many questions involved in a case like John's. There is more to it than genetics, or carcinogens in the environment. His cancer—and his cure—are involved with that "something else" of which I have spoken. To resolve the mystery, it becomes vital to search for other clues. In the cases of Jenny and John, and dozens of my other patients, a pattern can be discerned that links all these separate people together.

It is a pattern I first became aware of in the early 1950's, when I was working together with another research psychologist, Dr. Richard Worthington. On examining the personality tests of people who had later died of cancer, we found some startling similarities in their personality configurations and in their life histories. Worthington's suggestion that there might be a link between cancer and the ways in which the patient viewed himself and his world seemed to me a clue that must be tracked to earth.

For more than two decades I have been following the lead of that first clue. It has taken me far afield of the usual paths in cancer research. While doctors have long recognized that the personality and the emotions can cause such medical problems as ulcers, asthma and migraine headaches, there was strong resistance to the idea that there could be any psychosomatic basis for an organic disease so voracious as cancer. There were, after all, simple explanations for the development of ulcers in tense, anxious and over-worked individuals. Their tension caused the secretion of excess stomach acids, which ate away at the stomach lining, forming a lesion or ulcer. But how could a person's emotional state cause individual cells to alter their normal growth pattern and become malignant?

From the beginning, I knew that this question would be extremely difficult, if not impossible, to answer. Scientific *proof*, in which cause and effect can be unequivocally demonstrated, is hard to arrive at in any area involving the human personality. But the problem of demonstrable proof is one that plagues even the most controlled cancer experiments—which is why questions continue to be asked about laboratory research that produces cancer in animals through the ingestion or injection of suspected carcinogens.

Can the fact that large doses of a given chemical produce cancers in rats be convincingly extrapolated to prove that lesser amounts of the same chemical will inevitably produce cancer in humans, especially when exposure takes place over a far greater time span? There are doctors and researchers who say yes, and others who are skeptical. In regard to any theory that cannot be proved absolutely, questions will be raised. But cancer itself asks a question: life or death? Any theory, any approach, that holds the slightest possibility of increasing our understanding of the disease, not only should be investigated—it demands exploration.

Thus, I was determined to persevere, despite the fact that when I first began work on the question of a link between cancer and the emotions, I was turned away by one hospital and research center after another. The respected head of one cancer unit told me, "Even if in ten years you prove your theory, I won't believe it." Fortunately, this attitude has changed, not only in general, but in the case of this particular man. Recently, he was quoted in the *New York Times* as having "discovered" that certain personality characteristics were shared by his patients suffering from cancer. Developments in other areas of medicine, including evidence concerning the predisposition to heart attacks among high-strung "Type A" individuals, have given added respectability to the concept of psychosomatic involvement in life-threatening diseases.

In the course of my research, I discovered that in the 18th and 19th centuries the concept of a linkage between an individual's life history or personality and cancer was quite widely accepted. But why did this idea lapse into obscurity? There seem to be two possible reasons. To begin with, until Freud and other psychoanalytic pioneers began to develop the psychological tools with which to help people change the orientation of their personalities, there was little a doctor could do beyond merely observing the connection with emotional factors. Secondly, medical science has made great progress since the turn of the century in dealing with the purely physical aspects of cancer. Methods for early detection, improved surgical techniques, and new developments such as radiation and chemotherapy, have helped to save the lives of countless people. The success of these concrete technological methods of dealing with cancer has tended to foster a narrow focus on cancer as specifically located in one part of the body rather than opening the way to consideration of the whole person—in spite of the fact that psychological tools do now exist that make possible an alternate approach.

The success of surgical and other techniques certainly does not lessen the need for a further understanding of the psychological factors involved—not merely in respect to identifying emotional syndromes that may make certain individuals more susceptible to cancer, but also in helping those who are stricken to face the crisis in their lives in the most constructive way possible. An increasing number of doctors are expressing interest in why a patient who is expected to survive does not, and conversely, why another patient whose physical condition would seem to indicate an early death can continue to lead a full and satisfying life for many years. There is also increasing curiosity as to what lies behind the "miraculous" remissions that occur in some patients.

For all these reasons, I believe the time has arrived to explore these questions in a book intended for the general public. Drawing on more than two decades of my own research in this area, as well as upon the ongoing work by other researchers, physicians, and psychotherapists, my purpose is to explore three areas of central concern. First, I intend to set forth the extensive existing evidence that *there is a general type of personality configuration among the majority of cancer patients,* and to suggest some reasons why the emotional responses of these individuals make them more susceptible to cancer.

Secondly, and most importantly, I wish to outline a number of ways in which *people whose personality or life history conforms to this pattern of susceptibility can take steps to protect themselves against the possibility of cancer.* By developing a new outlook on their lives, and by being prepared to deal with certain kinds of emotional setbacks, I believe that potentially vulnerable individuals can create a degree of psychological "im-

12

munity" that will increase their chances of resisting the disease.

Finally, I will endeavor to show how the critically ill cancer patient can make the most of the remainder of his or her life. For the "terminal" patient, it is not a question of how many months or years of life remain, but how that time is to be lived. As a psychotherapist, I have treated many dozens of cancer patients over the years. In many cases it has been possible to help them achieve a sense of personal fulfillment they had never previously enjoyed, so that the period remaining to them became the most satisfying time of their lives. For some others who have responded fully to treatment, there has been a remission or stabilization of the cancer, and, like John the musician, they have happily survived for many years despite an initial diagnosis that appeared to leave them no hope.

Hope, in fact, is the true theme of this book. For it is the individual who, accepting his own being as valid, continually seeks self-fulfillment—the individual whose hopes for his own full rich life are sufficiently high to enable him to deal with temporary setbacks—who appears to be most resistant to cancer. Among those striken by the disease, the people most capable of recovery are the men and women who can discover a new well-spring of hope, whatever their past disappointments, and move on to a fresh sense of themselves, a true recognition of their needs, and of their worth as human beings.

The Search for a Pattern 2

When I began my research in the early 1950's, the modern literature on the subject of relationships between personality and cancer had not yet appeared. Most of the clinical reports pre-dating the twentieth century had been ignored for so long that their very existence had become obscured. Thus I found myself in a very real sense venturing into unknown territory. I was an explorer without maps; there were certain trails that seemed promising but I could not know whether they would truly lead me toward a broadening horizon or bring me up short in some morass of conflicting evidence.

Research into an area about which little is known poses special problems. It is not always feasible to formulate specific hypotheses and test them—that kind of approach must come later. Initially, the process must be of a more general investigative nature. One must look around in a variety of directions, attempt various methods of approach, gather as much information as possible, be vigilant for clues and relationships that hold the possibility of further exploration, and, not least, follow one's hunches. To organize concepts and test them according to the precise methods of science too early in the quest is likely to lead to sterility. Before formulating possible answers, one must learn enough to ask the right questions.

My first task, therefore, was to amass a large amount of material on the life history, the personality structure and the emotional functioning of patients with malignant disease. I would then study this material, evaluate it with respect to a variety of frames of reference, and generally "mull it over" to see what significant patterns might emerge. Using these first clues, I could look for similar patterns in other patients, as well as in control groups consisting of cancer-free individuals. Finally, if the patterns still appeared valid, I would go on to test them by classic scientific techniques.

In the first phase of this work—the gathering of material concerning the personality of cancer patients—three techniques were used. First, I gave a series of psychological tests to patients at the Institute of Applied Biology. By right of tradition in clinical psychology, the Rorschach ("ink-blot") Test appeared to be the best starting point. No other test has been so extensively used; no other is backed up by such a rich body of psychological literature. But certain difficulties arose.

The patients heard they were going to be given Rorschachs and talked about it among themselves before seeing their physicians. Because the Rorschach is such a well-known test, I had hoped that the patients would accept it as a matter of course. It was important that they not be told exactly why they were being asked to take the test—I did not want to arouse their anxiety, or to approach the test in terms of the fact that they had cancer, since that awareness might influence their choices.

Yet, unfortunately, a good deal of suspicion and resentment was apparent on the part of many of the patients. By and large, they were perplexed as to why they were being given a *psychological* test at all. The test results, or protocols, revealed both defensiveness and constriction. The clinic receptionist, who informally monitored the patients' discussions in the waiting room, made reports clearly indicating that the test was in fact arousing anxiety. This was the last thing I wanted, both in terms of getting valid information and in terms of the well-being of the patients.

There was a further problem. The Rorschach is in some ways a restricted test; it gives a great deal of information about the material in the subject's unconscious and good estimates of the strength and consistency of the ego. Except when used with exceptional skill, however, it gives much less data about how the patient functions in the world, how he has related to it in the past, and what his present day-to-day life is like. Yet it was exactly these concerns that seemed most important. If a link between personality and susceptibility to cancer were to be established, it seemed likely that it would show itself most clearly in the specific ways in which the individual lived in and related to his world, how he met the challenges of daily living, and how he viewed himself in terms of the on-going interaction between himself and the people and events of his life. Thus, only 30 Rorschachs of cancer patients were accumulated during the course of the study, although they did prove useful in helping to evaluate various elements of my hypothesis.

The next test to be tried was the Thematic Apperception Test (TAT). In this test, the patient is shown a series of pictures, of the typical magazine illustration type, and asked to make up a story as to what is happening in the picture. Although the TAT gives a broader picture of the personality of the patient, reactions to it were once again negative. It appeared that it would be very difficult to use the test on a large number of people without seriously impairing patient morale and without a large number of overt and covert refusals to be tested. A series of 15 TATs was obtained and during the later course of the research another 12 patients were given this test. These results also proved useful in making overall evaluations of the data.

Finally, another test was chosen that proved very

17

successful. This test, a life-history questionnaire called the Worthington Personal History, is a four-page information form that the patient fills out himself. It includes sections on such life-areas as family, schooling, work, hobbies, aims, goals, health, etc. In general, it resembles a typical vocational application form. Although not very well known, this test seemed admirably suited to the project. It gave an understanding of the major unconscious stresses, the ego defenses and the techniques of functioning and relating used in everyday life. It also gave a picture of where the patient had been in his life, what he had done and how he felt about different periods of his personal history. I was given access by Worthington Associates, Inc. to a group of 12,000 records taken from industrial studies, and these provided an excellent control group against which to measure the tests of cancer patients.

Of major importance was the fact that patients showed very little resistance to the test. Presented as "a form we would like to have you fill out so we can know more about you and be able to do a better job," the test aroused a minimum of anxiety, according to the evidence of discussions in the clinic waiting room. In the course of the study, 455 of these tests were given.

Another technique used for gathering fundamental information about the life situation and self-image of the cancer patient was the short interview. The form of these interviews had to be carefully considered. Structured interviews, in which a specific set of questions are asked of all those interviewed, present a special kind of problem, in that they delimit in advance the data that can be obtained. This, obviously, was unadvisable. The major difficulty of the early stages of my research was that it was impossible to know what data was being looked for. But unstructured interviews, on the other hand, can miss crucial life-areas.

A special factor to be dealt with was that the patient in a cancer service has to be given some reason why he is being interviewed. This reason does not have to be formally expressed, but the interview must "make sense" in a medical setting. Patients generally want to know why they are being interviewed or tested; and a superficial answer can arouse resentment that will lower the patient's morale and increase depressive feelings as well as contaminating the data that is elicited. Many patients are quite sensitive about the possibility of being treated as "guinea pigs" and care must be taken to avoid any semblance of doing so.

Furthermore, if no medical reason for the interview was apparent, patients would be likely to interpret it as a search for psychological factors in their illness. Since it has been shown that interviewees have a strong tendency to give the interviewer what he wants, severe distortions might well be introduced into the protocols. It was important to gain a picture of what the patient thought were pertinent factors in the development of his or her illness—but I recognized the danger of "suggesting" that psychological factors were indeed causative simply by the fact of giving a psychological examination. The patients, after all, were at the cancer center for *medical* treatment.

For these reasons, it was decided to start each interview with a history of the patient's illness. When had he first noted symptoms? What were they? How had he felt? What did he do? This had the added advantage of giving a picture of how the patient saw his illness *now*. Once the language the patient used in describing his own disease was understood, I could use the same terms, and thus avoid adding further stresses to the situation.

When this point was reached, I broadened the interview to include an occupational and geographical history of the patient's life. Thus, each interview began in a structured way, but as its focus widened, it became unstructured, and I left it to the patient to lead it in whatever direction he chose. Subsequently, a discussion of any major life-areas—childhood, schooling, hobbies—that had not been covered before concluded the interview. Because many cancer patients tire easily, the interview was broken into several sessions, and the patient was rarely kept for longer than an hour at a time.

In the course of my research, over a 14-year period, 250 patients were interviewed from 2 to 8 hours each. In addition, over two hundred cancer patients were given interviews or a series of interviews centered around any particular adjustment problem that they—or their physician—asked me to help them with. This "extra-curricular" series of interviews often helped my own understanding. And, as a kind of by-product of my work, I found myself seeing many relatives of cancer patients, who chiefly seemed to want someone they could ask questions of in order to reduce their own anxieties. It is tragic how often the relative of the cancer patient is left virtually alone with his or her problems. The patient has a peculiar horror all his own to live with, but the medical and auxiliary services of the hospital or clinic do furnish some support. Social workers equipped to aid relatives, however, are badly needed in most cancer institutions.

Close relatives of over 50 patients were interviewed for between one and three hours. An additional 40 close relatives were seen for between 20 and 50 hours. Often after a cancer patient had died, members of the family continued to come for psychological help for a considerable period. The opportunity to informally corroborate the patient's reports and to get another view of various aspects of his life was taken advantage of whenever possible. In most cases, the relatives seemed to obtain a good deal of relief helping in this informal process.

In the first two years of my research, only the psychological testing and the interviews were used as methods of gathering material on the subject. Later, when I felt that I had gained sufficient basic insight into the particular problems of cancer patients, I undertook the more complex and sensitive task of seeing many patients for intensive individual psychotherapy. Over 70 people eventually entered into such treatment. That later experience in most cases helped me further develop and sometimes alter my hypotheses concerning the relationship between cancer and personality that were developed in the first two years of the study. Before discussing the form of the individual psychotherapy sessions, however, I would like to set out in detail the patterns that emerged from the testing and interviewing carried out in the first two years.

As the test and interview protocols of the cancer patients were evaluated and compared, certain factors appeared to be present in record after record. The clues were indeed there.

The strongest clue concerned the loss of the patient's raison d'être (*literally, the "reason for being"*). This loss of their sense of purpose in life had occurred at some point in the past, apparently pre-dating the first noted symptoms of cancer. The Worthington Personal History test gives clues as to psychological functioning at different periods in the life of the subject. From the test and interview data, it appeared that for these patients who had lost their sense of purpose there had once been a period when they had participated much more fully in life. At that time they had had a relationship with a person or group that was of great and deep meaning to them. All other relationships had been comparatively superficial. The single central relationship satisfied their needs to express their creativity, to relate to others, to be a member of a group, to win response and recognition. Both their creative and their social needs had been expressed through the central relationship, and it was for them all-important. The exclusivity of such an intense single-minded relationship is beautifully expressed in the following lines from Shakespeare's *Othello*:

> . . . there where I have garned up my heart,
> Whether either I must live or bear no life,
> The fountain from which my current runs
> Or else dries up . . .

For these people, the loss of the central relationship can be catastrophic. The meaning and the validity of the individual's own life may be shattered. For these people, in Pericles's words, "The spring had gone out of the year." The loss of the crucial relationship naturally occurred through different circumstances with different patients. The death of a spouse, children growing up and becoming independent, the loss of a job, graduation from school—all appeared with some frequency. Often, there were indications that a major effort had been made to find substitute relationships, but these had failed and the patient remained deeply isolated even though he or she might be surrounded by family and friends. From a sociological point of view, the person had lost the only role that had real meaning to him.

On the surface, these people might seem to function in an adequate psychological manner, but underneath was an absence of direction or goal. They felt a lack of any stable reference points for themselves in the universe. There was no deep, solid emotional connection between the self and anything perceived outside of the self.

The fact that this loss of a central relationship, combined with the inability to establish new ones, appeared to be typical for the records of the cancer patients who were tested or interviewed, was clearly an important finding. It related directly to personality and to the way the patient saw himself in the world. But it also raised questions. Why had this one relationship meant so much to the patient? Why was it irreplaceable? What about the people who suffered similar losses but did *not* get cancer? What were the deeper meanings of the relationship to the patient? These and many other questions obviously needed to be asked, but the answers to them would have to await further study.

Other clues were also apparent in the early research. *The second of these was an inability on the part of the individual to express anger or resentment.* Frequently, these patients seemed to suppress and swallow their hostile feelings. They did have aggressive feelings, often quite strong ones, but they were unable to verbalize them. A façade of benign goodness was characteristic. Again, the reasons for this factor were not clear, but the immobilization of aggression appeared too frequently to be attributed to chance.

A third factor that seemed to statistically differentiate the cancer patients from the control group was the presence of indicators of emotional tension concerning the death of a parent. Often this death had occurred many years in the past, but continuing tension (apparently guilt or anxiety) was revealed on many of the test forms. In fact, however, this factor later proved to be a false clue, possibly the result of a sampling error. Further data, gathered later in the study, did not bear out its seeming significance.

Nevertheless, a start had been made. In order to further check on my hypothesis that the common factors I had found among the cancer patients might be connected with the incidence of the disease, I attempted to predict the presence of cancer in another group of individuals. Twenty-eight new Personal History records were obtained in such a way that I did not know which had been filled out by patients with malignant cancers and which by cancer-free individuals. None contained clues in the "health" area of the blank, or elsewhere, that would reveal the diagnosis. I knew only that "some" had been filled out by patients with malignancies. All were obtained by the receptionist at an out-patient medical clinic in Philadelphia.

The group of 28 Personal History Test records included 15 protocols of cancerous patients and 13 records of controls. The control group comprised 5 individuals with no known disease, 3 hyperthyroid persons, and one each with arteriosclerosis, allergy, psoriasis, dermatitis and obesity. The malignancies of the patients with cancer included 4 skin and 3 breast cancers, and one each of cancer of the thyroid, rectum, tongue, stomach, colon, uterus, cervix and the lymph nodes. Solely on the basis of the three psychological factors noted in this chapter,

TABLE I

Patients Evaluated in the First Phase of This Study

LOCATION OF MALIGNANCY	MALE	FEMALE	TOTAL
Breast	0	33	33
Colon and rectum	16	10	26
Buccal area	12	4	16
Skin	8	5	13
Lung	11	0	11
Stomach	6	2	8
Uterus	0	8	8
Hodgkin's disease	6	1	7
Cervix	0	6	6
Miscellaneous	18	6	24
Total number of patients (N)	77	75	152

TABLE II

The Psychological Factors Found

FACTOR	CANCER PATIENTS N—152	CONTROLS N—125
Loss of a crucial relationship	109 (72%)	15 (12%)
Inability to express hostility	71 (47%)	31 (25%)
Tension over death of a parent	58 (38%)	13 (11%)

I attempted to predict which patients had cancer and which did not.

My predictions were correct in 24 out of the 28 cases. Three non-cancerous patients, one with arteriosclerosis, one with allergy, and one with hyperthyroidism were predicted to have cancer. One patient with cancer of the skin was predicted as being unaffected. Statistically, the probability that this number of correct predictions would occur by chance is less than one in a thousand.

Thus, I felt confident that the study was moving in the right direction. In this first phase, the records of 152 cancer patients had been studied. A control series (equated by age, sex and social class) of 125 subjects with no known disease had also been evaluated. All records were of subjects who, judged by occupational status, were of upper-lower or middle class. Tables I and II show the kinds of malignancy suffered by these patients and the psychological factors found. Clearly, the loss of a crucial relationship, which had occurred in the lives of 72% of the patients, was the most significant clue in my search for possible relationships between the life history of the individual and a vulnerability to cancer. Both this factor and the second most prevalent one—the inability to express hostility—were to take on additional meaning in the next phase of my work, which was to involve intensive individual psychotherapy. As we shall see in the next chapter, this new phase provided both a fresh perspective and a much deeper understanding of the significance of the factors already uncovered.

A Fuller Picture Emerges 3

The data of the projective test protocols and that of the short interview series conducted during the first phase of my research seemed to agree. A definite pattern had presented itself, a pattern sufficiently clear so that it was possible to predict the existence of cancer in an individual with considerable accuracy, based only upon personality tests. Yet the pattern was merely an outline.

An artist painting a portrait of a particular human being may begin by drawing an outline of the person's head and shoulders. While those initial lines upon the canvas may be recognizable in a rudimentary way, it is not until the specific features have been filled in—the way the lips curl in a smile, the slight flare of a nostril, the expression of the eyes—that a fully significant picture of the unique human being will begin to emerge. Thus, in the next phase of my work, through in-depth psychotherapeutic exploration with particular individuals, I hoped and expected that greater richness and meaning would be given to my rather bald original findings.

The factors already uncovered seemed to be amenable to statistical treatment, but statistics are only pegs upon which to hang a fuller, more rounded picture. The rich tapestry that each human being is, many-colored and marvelously woven, can easily be lost in a table of figures. If the validity of the factors I had already noted was to be sustained, they would have to make sense within the more explicit context of the particular life histories of individuals about whom I knew a great deal more than can be inferred from a test or an interview lasting a few hours.

Psychotherapy today is a term that covers a wide variety of techniques. These range from Rogerian non-directive practices, through formal psychoanalysis to extremely directive methodologies. The question of what approach would be best, in terms both of the patient and my own research, was a difficult one. Obviously, some methods were automatically excluded because I had not received formal training in them—the Jungian and Adlerian disciplines, for instance. An orthodox psychoanalytic approach appeared questionable. However admirably suited it may be to the understanding and solution of some neurotic problems, it did not seem suitable to dealing with the realities that must be faced by a cancer patient. Full responsibility to the subjects had to be recognized in the method chosen, and the psychotherapy had to be of a genuine sort, not just for research purposes. Over a twelve-year period, I devised such a method and worked with it further over an additional ten years. It is described in depth in a later chapter, but at this point it is of more immediate concern to describe the further clues that were discovered in respect to the link between the emotions and cancer.

In the course of twenty-two years, 70 patients with terminal malignancies underwent intensive psychotherapy with me. All but one were aware of their diagnosis and of the usual prognosis for their type of disease before the therapy started. Eighty-eight patients without known malignancies were treated by means of the same therapeutic technique. These patients, of the kind usually seen in office practice of psychotherapy, provided me with a control group, making it possible to ascertain whether or not the factors that seemed particularly significant in cancer victims were indeed more prevalent among people who contracted the disease.

The selection of patients for therapy was a somewhat haphazard affair—how could one know in advance what types of cancer patients should be given psychotherapy? Usually, their selection grew out of the short interview series. Patients who seemed in the interviews to be good therapy subjects, and who expressed a desire to go on, were told of the opportunity. In all cases but one they accepted. Fifteen patients heard about the therapy program on the hospital grapevine or through friends, and personally requested that they be taken on. Two patients were old friends of mine. (When I heard that one of them had a malignancy that could not be treated by medical means, I flew down to his home town and offered him the opportunity.) Five patients came to me as the result of reading about the therapy in scientific journals. One patient was referred to me by a local Mental Hygiene Clinic. And five patients were originally referred to me for supportive therapy, which later developed into intensive psychotherapy.

Objections can no doubt be raised that the selection of these patients was not sufficiently random for research of this kind. As a group their average age was younger than a statistically random selection would have decreed. There was a heavy emphasis on Hodgkin's disease (12 patients); and all were in the upper quartile of the intelligence curve. But in a small group—as this had to be since there are limitations to the number of patients one therapist can see—randomization must be carefully planned. And which of the thousands of potentially crucial variables would one randomize? Since the results of my own research have been largely corroborated by other later studies (see Chapter Five), objections concerning the makeup of the group I worked with would appear to be moot.

As noted in the first chapter, it was difficult to find a facility in which this research program could be carried out. Fifteen major hospitals turned me down on the grounds that they had had no space available or, more frequently, because the hospital did not care to be associated with research into the area. It was often stated that even to *investigate* this area was the approach of a charlatan! The reasons behind this blatantly close-minded reaction have never been clear to me. And while this reaction was common among medically trained personnel, it has never, to my knowledge, been voiced by an actual cancer patient. Fortunately this attitude has changed, and a number of similar research programs have been started in recent years at various major hospitals and clinical centers. As for my own work, an excellent and stimulating arrangement was made with the Institute of Applied Biology, in New York City, and it was there that the full picture of the personality of the cancer patient gradually unfolded.

The first clues provided by the psychotherapy concerned two new factors and a modification of one previously observed. As these new factors were suggested by the psychotherapy, the protocols of the tests and the interview series were re-evaluated accordingly.

One new factor was a marked amount of self-dislike and self-distrust observed in these cancer patients. These individuals did not respect their own accomplishments; they did not like themselves or the attributes they perceived in themselves. In a majority of cases, they had basically accepted (and often over-compensated for) self-perceptions such as "stupid," "lazy," "mediocre," "destructive," etc. Other people responded to them much more positively than they did to themselves, but this, of course, took none of the sting out of their beliefs about themselves.

This factor could, of course, also apply to many neurotics. Karen Horney in particular has described in detail this type of self-feeling. However, both its frequency and its strength among the cancer patients was notable. One young woman, for instance, compared herself to Rappaccini's Daughter, in the story by Hawthorne. "I need love and can respond to love," she said, "but I poison them [anyone she loves] because they don't have my immunity to my own poison." Statements of this kind among the cancer patients seemed to go beyond the usual self-rejection of the neurotic. Indeed, as we shall see, they tie in with other factors typical of the personality of the cancer patient.

The psychotherapy also led to a modification of one factor observed earlier—the inability to express hostility. It became clear that these patients were frequently blocked in their ability to express hostility in their own defense, but that they could stand strongly and aggressively in defense of the rights of others or of ideals. Thus it was not a general inability to become aggressive, but rather an inability to become aggressive in terms of their own needs, wishes and feelings. They did not see their own desires as justifying defense.

Karen Horney has stated a basic equation of the neurotic: "I am unrelated to others as if I were a comet flying through space. Therefore, the wishes and needs of others have no validity." But while the cancer patient feels a similar isolation, his or her conclusion is entirely different: "Therefore *my* wishes have no validity." Frequently, I found, the cancer patient's own desires and wishes had been so completely repressed, and the self-alienation was so total that when at the start of therapy I asked the question, "What do *you* really want out of life?" the response would be a blank and astonished stare. That question had never been seen as valid.

Both the self-alienation and the inability to become aggressive in their own defense were factors strongly related to an even more important—in fact fundamental —feeling about life that characterized the cancer patients. This basic element in the emotional life of the cancer patient I call "despair." It was observed in 68 out of the 71 therapy patients studied—yet it was found in only three of the control group of 88.

It should be made clear from the outset that this despair was not a result of having contracted cancer. It was rather a fundamental aspect of the patients' emotional makeup, a feeling they had lived with all their lives. To make the point even more strongly, many of the patients specifically expressed the idea that for years they had felt there was no way out of the emotional box they found themselves in short of death itself.

As observed in the emotional life of cancer patients, "despair" appeared to be a basic *Weltanschauung,* or "world-view," with three secondary components. The central orientation appeared to be a bleak hopelessness about ever achieving any meaning, zest or validity in life. This is a much more barren and hopeless outlook than that expressed by the usual depressed patient. The alienation felt by the "normal" depressed, suicidal or otherwise self-destructive patient often allows a continued contact with others, even if it is composed primarily and consciously of hostile rather than loving elements. The despair of the cancer patient, on the other hand, brings about a sense of aloneness that makes it impossible not only for love to bridge the gap, but also excludes the possibility of fully and satisfyingly relating to others even in terms of anger, resentment or jealousy.

The patient in despair is absolutely alone. At the deepest emotional level he cannot relate, since he does not believe himself worthy of love. He does not despair over "something," as would the usual depressed patient —rather, he despairs over "nothing." After a patient had expressed some negative feelings about herself, I asked her, "What do you think it is that makes you so angry at yourself—that makes you feel so guilty? Do you feel you have done something to deserve this?" And she replied, "No, I've done nothing. You don't understand, doctor. It's not that I've been or done anything. It's that I've done *nothing* and been *nothing*."

It was statements such as these that made me begin to understand that the central task of psychotherapy where the cancer patient is concerned must be finding and celebrating the full individuality of the patient. How this can be done—and it can—is a subject that we will be returning to again and again throughout this book.

As the intensive therapy sessions continued, I was able with the help of some concepts of Edgar N. Jackson, to isolate three secondary components of the cancer patient's despair. First, there is a lack of belief that outside "objects" can bring satisfaction. Any meaning achieved through relating, the patient feels, can only be —at best—temporary, and inevitably will bring disappointment and pain. Secondly, there is an absence of faith in development. There is no belief that either time or the patient's own development can change his basic condition of life. Individuals who are not in despair always see the possibility of growth or change affecting the painful condition in a positive way. The person in despair simply does not see this as a possibility. There is, thirdly, an absence of belief that any action the patient takes can ease his aloneness. To be what he is, is to be rejected. No amount of effort can change this. Generally, major efforts have been made by the patient —often gigantic amounts of energy have been poured into attempts to reach others. But these efforts have failed and seemed doomed to fail eternally, from that patient's point of view.

It is difficult to give clear examples of despair, as expressed in the particular words of given patients. The feeling emerges slowly, at many times and in changing forms. But a few examples may give some indication of the overall feeling.

"It's as if all my life I've been climbing a very steep mountain. It's very hard work. Every now and then there are ledges I can rest on and even enjoy myself for a little while. But I've got to keep climbing. And the mountain I'm on has no top."

"I found I hated working for the union. It was too late to go back to music, although I tried. I knew I'd have to stay in the business end for good. There was no way out, no matter what I did."

"The more I tried to tear it down, the higher and thicker became the wall of thorns I had built around myself. I couldn't get past it to other people. I feel like Dornrosen [the fairy tale princess who slept inside a circle of thorns until a prince breached it and awakened her] except that the forest has grown so thick that no one will find me. The path is too overgrown ever to be used again."

"No matter what I did, it didn't work. I lost my ability (to write) and so did Tom, and the more we tried, the worse it got. I gave up everything for him—I see it now —it destroyed us both. We had a mutual strangulation society. There just didn't seem any way out . . . I often thought I'd only escape by dying."

"You know how it is with a house with no insulation and with cracks in the walls. The more you put in heat, the more it leaks out. You can never get warm. I always knew that's how it was with me in life. I had to keep putting out, and there was never any reflection back at me. If I was going to get warm inside, I'd have to do it alone, and no matter how much you do, you can't do that."

A house with no insulation.

A mountain with no top.

A path too overgrown ever to be used again.

No way out.

An escape only in dying.

Listening to this litany of despair, certain questions came back to me over and over again.

How could these cancer victims be helped to regain a sense of their own worth, of the possibilities of growth and change in themselves and their relationships?

If such a renewal could be achieved, was it possible that some of them—a few or many—could go on living far beyond the short time given to them by purely medical determination?

What of the thousands of individuals who had not yet contracted cancer, but whose lives were clouded by the same hopelessness? Could they be helped? And if they could, might the onslaught of cancer be delayed or avoided?

The patients I was seeing were, by my own choice, people who were given no chance of survival. Their malignancies were terminal. But what of those who developed cancer and survived? What resources did they bring to their battle for life that my patients lacked?

Answers to all these questions began to appear, bit by bit. Some of the answers were partial ones. None was absolute. Yet, as my work went on, I came to believe more and more completely that my original hypothesis had been correct: there *was* a link between personality and cancer. And the more thoroughly that link came to be understood, by myself and by others who might follow, the greater was the possibility of reducing the risk of cancer for countless human beings. For whatever the depth of despair of any individual patient, I knew that change was possible, that a man or woman can come to see his or her life in a new, more rational and hopeful light. Not every individual could be helped. But some could. And the example of those who did achieve a fresh outlook would make it possible to convince still others that hope was never dead.

In most of my patients, psychotherapeutic exploration revealed that their despairing orientation had remained unverbalized until the therapy clarified it. It also showed that their despair had existed prior to the first signs of a tumor. Despite their feelings about life, these people had functioned in their daily existence, had continued the routine work of their lives, even though they had never believed that life could hold any satisfaction for them. Only the Dark Bridegroom, death itself, could offer eventual surcease from the otherwise endless necessity of working at the impossible. Each of them had followed in the footsteps of the mythical Sisyphus—rolling the stone constantly up the hill, knowing they could not reach the top, but having to keep on trying.

Most of my patients had repressed the emotions connected with despair. They accepted their lives as they saw them with a stoic lack of bitterness or resentment. Elizabeth Barrett Browning's poem "Grief" well expresses the quality of such lives:

I tell you, hopeless grief is passionless;
   That only men incredulous of despair
   Half-taught in anguish, through the midnight air
Beat upward to God's throne in loud access
of shrieking and reproach. Full desertness,
   In souls as countries, lieth silent-bare
   Under the blanching, vertical eye-glare
Of the absolute heavens.

The fact that the patient feels that there can be no
hope of solving his problem by his actions seems to be
an extremely important element. In his deep and wise
exploration of this psychological problem, the philosopher Kierkegaard points out that to get rid of one's
despair, one must get rid of one's self—the self that
one despairs of. But to be rid of one's self is also a
cause of despair, since it means no longer to be one's
self. This is a concept that cancer patients advance again
and again. They feel that they can be themselves—and
therefore unloved and alone—or, that they can get rid
of themselves to be someone else and thus be loved.
To them it appears that these are the only paths open.

One patient, in expressing this feeling, saw it as a
conflict between her "individuality" and her "popular-
ity." This young woman, Alma, went on to say, "It's
as if I have to have both food and water to live and
I can only have one of them." To give up her individuality, her own way of seeing and reaching the world,
meant the loss of herself; but to retain it meant to be
alone.

There is an important difference here between how the neurotic and the patient in despair view change in themselves. The neurotic may not wish to change himself and may show strong resistance to doing so, but it never occurs to him that if he *does* change he will be anyone but himself. The patient in despair, on the other hand, believes that if he changes he will inevitably cease to be an individual. If he changes, in his view, he will have annihilated himself. In this sense, his despair seems to him justified. He sees himself as being in the trap of having to exist in the present unbearable isolation or not existing at all. Once again, it should be emphasized that this view of the world *pre-dates* the development of the cancer.

Alma, the young woman quoted above, was a brilliant, highly trained specialist in her field. Yet early in therapy, she expressed a great deal of anxiety about being a "mediocrity," an everyday type of person with no special features. This anxiety seemed an example of the self-contempt noted previously as part of the makeup of the cancer patient. Yet there seemed to be more to it than that. Further exploration revealed that she knew herself to be unusual, and that she in fact feared giving in to her own need to *become* a mediocrity deliberately, to give up her special differences in order to try to win love and acceptance. Despite her fears that she would do this, Alma was never able to accept the "Faustian" bargain; she retained her sense of individuality, and with it her aloneness.

Another patient, Stephen, stated in his first session

that he had always been an independent person, who had "never needed a pillow" in his life. The qualities of strength, competence, dominance and independence marked the central parts, the bone structure, of his individuality, according to his own view of himself. As the therapy progressed, however, it developed that he felt he could not be loved as himself. He felt that as himself he could gain only fear and respect, and that in order to inspire the love he so desperately needed, he would have to become passive, dependent and weak. He, like Alma, could not make this bargain; yet he felt that he could not gain what he needed otherwise. He could neither express nor reject his passive and dependent needs. While he could not conceive of accepting the dependent part of himself sufficiently to allow it a natural outlet, he nevertheless was aware, in some dim fashion, that until he could do so he would not be whole, would indeed be rejecting a basic part of himself. Expending more and more energy in a frenzied attempt to gain love through domination and control—an attempt he knew must fail and yet felt compelled to continue—he deeply wished only to die, so that he would be able to cease the struggle.

Emily had many of the same conflicts as Alma and Stephen, but went further in attempting to divest herself of her "individuality." Since childhood, Emily had had an intense drive to write poetry. Her view of herself and her reactions to the world around her were seen within this frame of reference. Her work was of a very high and unusual quality, but she was unable to show it to anyone but her husband. She had never submitted any of it for publication. She felt it would reveal how different she was from everyone else and would cause her to be rejected by others. It was only after several months of therapy that—with much anxiety—she showed some of her work to me. I privately obtained a professional opinion of it, which corroborated my own impression that it was of the first rank.

Emily had married a writer and for a brief time the relationship had been positive and intense. Her husband, Tom, was just beginning his career and felt confident of his future development. When it became apparent that her own abilities were far greater than anything Tom could expect of his own potential, her writing became a real threat to him, and he withdrew emotionally from their relationship. She felt that her early anxieties about whether to be a poet or to be loved were now justified by reality. (While the neurotic would see the choice as one of being a poet or a housewife, Emily viewed it as a matter of being a poet or nothing.) She tried to give up her poetry, tried very hard to give up all of herself to Tom. However, the relationship did not improve, and she found herself unable either to write *or* to be loved, and was deeply despairing of any real satisfaction in her life. Subsequently, her malignancy was discovered.

In practically all of my patients, some formulation of this dilemma was found. They all felt, to one degree or another, that to gain what they needed to bring meaning to their lives, they must give up themselves and become something else. Even to consider this solution gave rise to despair. To accomplish it, for any length of time, was impossible. As might have been predicted, giving up themselves and attempting to be someone or something else did not in fact win the love they so desperately sought. Most had tried and succeeded for a period of time in denying what they saw as their "true" selves. But sooner or later the attempts broke down. While they were actually involved in the attempt, their despair had, of course, intensified. Basically, they could not accept the idea of winning love at the cost of their perceived selves. Like Joan of Arc in Jean Anouilh's *The Lark*, they found themselves saying, "What I am, I will not denounce; what I have been, I will not deny."

To some, the dilemma of these individuals may seem perverse, even incomprehensible. How can anyone think that way? How can anyone paint himself into such a corner? Yet this view of the self is held by countless human beings. It is a theme that has been articulated in the literature of mankind down through the ages. The Greek playwright Aeschylus, whose works are among the most ancient surviving expressions of the human condition, is deeply expressive of this dilemma. Aeschylus's great triology, *The Oresteia*, presents the theme in the clearest possible terms. Should Orestes obey Apollo (reason, logic, custom, law) and thus be pursued by the Furies (the earth spirit, the instinctive part of the human being, the inner self, the soul)? Or should he obey the dictates of the Furies and thus disobey and disavow

Apollo? Aeschylus sees that there is a possible integration of these two aspects, which are synthesized through the intervention of the goddess Athena in the final play of the trilogy, *The Eumenides*. But such an integration, such a synthesis, simply does not occur to the cancer patients I have studied. They do not regard it as conceivable.

The dilemma is also embodied in Hermann Hesse's great novel of existential despair, *Steppenwolf*. Harry Haller, the protagonist, sees himself as two separate personalities in one body: the civilized man and the wolf of the steppes. He believes suicide to be the only way out; only death will offer him release from the terrible struggle between the two aspects of himself. It is a struggle made hopeless by his perception that victory for either aspect means the destruction of the other, thus sundering the totality, the whole self of Haller. And yet, in his conception, the two cannot coexist, although a temporary truce can sometimes be achieved. The statement of the problem in this novel, as well as the solution that Hesse presents, can be of great value in conveying to the despairing patient the nature of his condition. Indeed, Hesse's solution clearly outlines much that must happen in successful psychotherapy with these individuals—a subject we will be returning to later.

Alma, Stephen, Emily, indeed all my patients, related their despair only superficially to their cancers. Their fatal disease was seen only as "one more example" of the hopelessness of life for them. They stated that they had felt despairing long before the disease made itself known. The fact that they had become fatally ill merely confirmed what they already believed about themselves —that their situation had never afforded any hope. The problem of their unbearable existence was in fact being solved for them by the cancer—finally, and irrevocably, they were getting rid of themselves. This was the solution that they had always figuratively feared and yet felt to be inescapable.

Their despair did not seem to be a symptom of psychotherapeutic resistance. Rather, it appeared to be an uncovering of something already there, making overt what had been covert. But in view of this orientation, it had to be asked why the patients continued to go on with the routine of their daily existence? And, in addition, how could they relate to their therapist?

Let me offer some tentative answers to these questions. The patients appeared to be willing to "go on," in spite of their beliefs that they would accomplish nothing of real meaning, exactly because they were able to perceive only two possible paths for themselves. The choice lay only between being "themselves" and being "someone else." The "either-or" view of the cancer patient seems to press him to continue his accustomed activities as long as these are physically possible. One clear difference between despair and depression lies in this area. The depressed patient does *not* go on with his usual activities—the greater the depression, the greater the tendency to give them up. But the patient in despair shows no tendency to slow down; he keeps on at his usual pace. No matter how acute the despair, routine activities of daily life are maintained.

One might expect that, faced with a sentence of death, these patients would attempt to have new experiences, or fulfill old dreams. But this reaction is in fact startlingly rare. Suicide also is rare, unless the pain becomes overwhelming. While many of these patients spoke of death as the only way out, they seemed willing to let the cancer run its course. The possibility of suicide had always existed in the past, but been put aside or repressed. Menninger has reported on three elements in the suicidal patient: the wish to die; the wish to kill; the wish to be killed. In the person in despair, only the wish to die seems to be present. Also lacking is the aggression against others that is often a component of the act of suicide. Thus the cancer patient, certain that the end will come as he has always felt it would, simply continues with his life as he has always lived it.

However, there is one important change that takes place in cancer patients after they learn of the presence of their malignancy: psychotherapy becomes generally acceptable to them, while in most cases it was not before. One might hypothesize that, once the choice of existence or non-existence has been made for them by the disease process, some psychic energy formerly bound up in their conflict is released. Only after the choice has been made for them are they able to dimly perceive the possibility of the middle road that the therapist offers. It is known in social work that the best time to start therapy with juvenile delinquents is often at the point of their first commitment to an institution or treatment center. The recognition that they are at the final dead end of one road seems to free them for the first time to consider whether there might be other roads. A similar process appears to be operating in cancer patients.

The remarkable results that can be achieved with some patients—including in several cases a startling remission of the cancer itself, even though the patient had been considered terminal—will be discussed in later chapters. In the next chapter, however, drawing upon what I learned from the test protocols, the interviews, and the intensive psychotherapy sessions, I will present a generalized life history of the typical cancer patient, drawing together the various themes that have been touched upon so far.

The Emotional Life History of Cancer Patients 4

One of my patients, Catherine, was a 32-year-old woman suffering from Hodgkin's disease, a form of cancer that affects the lymph glands. She had not been a happy child, and had felt rejected and unloved. Her mother had been an intellectually driven woman who dominated Catherine's submissive father. There was a sister, two years younger than Catherine, who was "the beauty" of the family. Attempts to get love from her mother seemed to result only in anger, since they interfered with the mother's social and political interests. The father, who had a strong puritanical background, regarded any physical contact with his daughter as repugnant. And Catherine felt unable to compete in attractiveness with her sister. Her one interest was music. She greatly enjoyed her piano lessons, showing unusual talent. Retreating from the whirl of her family's extensive social life, she preferred to go to her room alone to practice or to read biographies of great musicians.

The emotional pattern of Catherine's childhood was typical of my cancer patients. In almost all cases, damage had been done to the child's developing ability to relate early in life, usually during the first seven years. From their experience at this time, these children, who many years later would become cancer victims, learned to feel that emotional relationships brought pain and desertion. They were to be invested in deeply only at the cost of much pain and rejection. Loneliness became the child's doom. In the usual manner of children, their loneliness was attributed to some fault in themselves, rather than to accidental forces or the actions of others. Guilt and self-condemnation were the inevitable response.

In some cases, the sense of rejection was accentuated by a specific event. Richard, for instance, who developed Hodgkin's disease when he was 24, had been strongly affected by the death of his father. Richard had been only five at the time, yet he had felt in some undefined way responsible for his father's death, and for the economic pressures that subsequently afflicted his family. The fact that his mother had been pregnant with another child at the time of his father's death increased Richard's sense of being terribly alone.

The traumatic situation or crisis that affected these children usually did not have the kind of intensity that was likely to produce obvious neurotic symptoms. On the surface, the child would manage to adjust adequately to his or her environment. Yet the child's belief that social relationships were dangerous and that there was something wrong with himself persisted and colored his entire life. Little real energy was invested in relationships. The child was usually a "loner," with few friends. The relationships that were developed were usually superficial. And no matter what these children achieved —good grades, the development of an artistic ability— their basic feelings of failure predominated.

At some time in their development, however, usually in late adolescence or early adulthood, a situation would arise that offered these individuals an opportunity for relating to others. There was a perceived chance to end the deep loneliness that they felt. Richard, for instance, had occupied himself as a child with a deep interest in science. In high school, he joined various science clubs, which gave him the opportunity to relate to others in terms of his one true passion in life. By his junior year, he had become a fully accepted member of a group of students who worked together on various scientific experiments. Richard joined these friends every afternoon at club meetings, and spent the evenings in their cellar laboratories. He was never tired, and seemed to have plenty of time for schoolwork, for his hobbies, and for the afternoon and weekend jobs he held during most of this period. He felt truly "alive," involved completely in what he was doing, and full of hope for the future, planning to become an engineer.

Catherine, on the other hand, did not open herself up to the possibility of this kind of commitment, and the relationships it involved, until she was somewhat older. Her first year away at college had been lonely and unhappy. She did poorly in her studies, had no friends except her music teacher, and as final examinations approached, became tense and terrified. The evening before the first examination she slipped on the sidewalk and badly fractured her shoulder. Instead of returning to college, she persuaded her family (with the help of her mother's psychotherapist) to permit her to study piano in another city. It was there that she began to become involved in life in a new way.

She took an apartment with two other girls who were studying art and music, and the three of them became close friends. They worked hard at their studies and at practicing, and spent long hours talking and exploring the city. "I felt as if new doors were opening to me every day," she said in describing this period. "It was a *wonderful* year. I still feel nostalgic about it." For the first time, Catherine began dating, at first with men to whom she was introduced by the other girls. She loved her work. "I knew I could be a great pianist. I would often practice eight or ten hours a day, and we'd go to a concert or walk around the city and end up in a restaurant or eating in our rooms. We'd talk all night, and the next day I'd be ready to start all over again."

Both Richard and Catherine poured a tremendous amount of psychic and physical energy into these happy times of their lives. It was as though all the need for warm and intense relating that had been unexpressed for years was being released all at once. This intense emotional involvement was typical of my cancer patients during that period in their lives when they were able— for a while—to develop relationships that gave them a sense of life's meaningfulness. Their feelings of isolation and "lostness" were greatly eased by their new-found involvement. The relationship or relationships entered into at this time became the central focus of their lives —the *raison d'être*. Other relationships and channels of expression and creativity were usually maintained, but they continued to be somewhat superficial, and peripheral to the real core of their beings. In a sense, having at last found an outlet for their emotions, they tended to put all their eggs into one basket. All meaning, all creativity, all happiness was seen as being bound up in this particular situation or relationship.

When the situation changed, or the relationships faltered, it was all the more devastating to these people because they had invested themselves so completely in this one possibility for happiness. To be deprived of these relationships was to be deprived of *everything*, to fall back totally into the old loneliness, a loneliness compounded by the fear of further loss.

The period of involvement for these individuals often

53

ended through circumstances over which they had no control or felt that they didn't. In Richard's case, for instance, he felt that after graduating from high school he had a responsibility to support his mother, since she had worked so hard to keep him in school. The plans he had made to become an engineer were reluctantly abandoned, and he took a well-paid job as a truck driver. Richard tried to keep up his scientific interests, but he was unable to maintain his contacts with the friends he had made in high school, most of whom went on to college. For a while, he pursued his experiments alone, but his working hours were long and irregular, and both his energy and his interest began to flag. As time went on, his life came to seem less and less rewarding. Even the fact that he was bringing home money and helping his family brought him no real sense of satisfaction. His feeling of isolation was increased by the fact that his fellow truck drivers did not accept him. And four years after graduating from high school, Richard learned that he had the first symptoms of Hodgkin's disease.

Catherine's plans also did not go as she had wished. She and the other two girls she had lived with planned to return to the same apartment after the summer and continue their studies. But Catherine's father told her that she could not return, that life in the big city was too "immoral," and that he would not have his daughter living a "life of that kind." He finally convinced her that she would be just as happy at a small progressive college, and she consented to change her plans. But she felt unhappy and depressed at the new school. Her interest in music diminished. "Although I kept practicing," she told me, "my music was cold, there was nothing of *me* in it any more."

Catherine met a rather emotionally disturbed man whom she quickly married. On her first view of him through a window, she had said to a friend, "That's the man my mother would like me to marry." Despite Ted's inability to earn a living, they had four children in rapid succession. Catherine desperately tried to build a strong emotional relationship with Ted but, like her father, he was afraid of his own warm impulses, and the harder she tried to develop a closeness between them, the less he was able to respond.

Catherine also tried to form close friendships with other young women, but couldn't stand their constant talk of children and homes, while they quickly wearied of her attempts to talk of music, art and social issues. Although she joined a chamber music group, the demands of her family made it impossible for her to spend much time on her music. She found herself becoming more and more easily fatigued and increasingly less interested in anything. Her piano playing continued to become less satisfying. She felt that she would never succeed at anything or get any real enjoyment out of life. Within eight years, she too was a victim of Hodgkin's disease.

In some cases, the central relationship of these patients' lives was sustained over a long period of time.

Yet the emotional pattern of these individuals was marked by the same characteristics found in those for whom the central relationship was brief. Arthur, a patient with lung cancer, was 54 years old. During his early childhood, he had experienced a warm family life, but then when Arthur was four, his father deserted the home. Arthur felt hostile toward his father, but also guilty at having this reaction. Lacking feelings of support—which he had originally received from his father —he concentrated all his energy in work, first in school and later in the business world. He gained a considerable degree of security from material success, yet always felt that something was lacking in his life. His relationships with others, including his wife and child, were superficial, but his relationship with his job was not. He loved his work and put an immense amount of drive and fervor into it. He would work and see clients and colleagues all day, while drinking heavily in the evenings. The next morning, with very little sleep, he would be bright and active. I interviewed some of his co-workers from this period of his life, and they all corroborated the intensity of his energy, as well as his remarkable ability to organize major industrial campaigns despite his evening carousing and lack of sleep.

After achieving a very high level of occupational success, he was offered at the age of 49 a new job by an easy-going and kindly man. Arthur saw this man as "being the balance I'd always needed." Becoming this man's friend and follower, Arthur suppressed his own initiative and drive. He gave up drinking and joined A.A.

But gradually, he came to realize that his superior was in reality somewhat inefficient and undependable. Arthur rationalized his immobilization and remained on the job. But his energy output became blocked, and was considerably lowered. For years he had been working very hard; now he found himself able to carry out only the most routine tasks. For the first time in his life he felt bored. At the same time he became more and more hostile toward his superior, but did not give expression to his feelings. His devotion to his work disappeared and he was left without an outlet for his energy. He tried to occupy himself by giving more time to his family, and by working with A.A. and church groups. But these activities brought him little satisfaction. His demoralized and stultifying condition continued for two years before the lung cancer appeared.

The expenditure of energy—not just physical energy but psychic or emotional energy—during the periods when these cancer patients were able to relate to the world in a sustained way is in marked contrast to their sense of lassitude when they were subsequently deprived of that relationship. And in this contrast lies a vital clue to our understanding of the emotional life history of cancer victims. In all the cancer patients seen during the course of my research—over 500—not a single one seemed to me to have access to more emotional expression than he had energy to express. All seemed to have more emotional energy than they had ways of expressing it. Typically, there was a "bottled-up" quality to their emotional lives. This was not true, however, for the control subjects who did not have cancer. In fact, among the control patients it was common for them to be faced with *more* demands than they had energy.

The lack of ways in which to express their emotional energy, and indeed their inability to express it, affected the cancer patients in two ways. First, as we have seen previously, these individuals were unable to give vent to their feelings, to let other people know when they felt hurt, angry or hostile. Time and time again, in the test protocols, the short interviews, and the intensive psychotherapy sessions, it was clear that the cancer patients had difficulty in showing anger or aggression in defense of themselves. Other people would say, "She's a saint," or, "He's such a good, sweet man." Yet the benign quality, the "goodness" of these people was in fact a sign of their failure to believe in themselves sufficiently, and of their lack of hope. Seeing themselves as worthless, and their lives without meaning, they simply could not bring themselves to believe that they might be right in a given situation, and the other person wrong.

A number of years after I began my own research, a psychological appraisal was made by Dr. David Kissen of over 300 patients at a chest clinic. Half of the patients were subsequently found to be suffering from lung cancer. The remaining half served as a control group. Kissen found that there was a personality characteristic that differentiated the two groups from one another. Those with what he described as "a poor outlet for emotional discharge" were much more likely to have cancer. Further study showed that the lung cancer mortality rate (per 100,000 persons a year), was 270 for those with a poor outlet, but only 59 for those with a good outlet. This difference existed, significantly, at all levels of cigarette smoking.

The importance of emotional outlets—or the lack of them—can be shown not only by such statistical analysis; it can also be dramatically seen in individual case histories. One of my patients, Louise, was a 60-year-old woman with breast cancer. As a young child, she had been much loved and protected. The family was European, but when Louise was seven, her father left home to come to America. He took the older children with him, and the family was split for several years. Repressing her hostility toward her father, and her sense of loss, she changed her role and became an "assistant mother," thus denying her own need for protection. As a life pattern she has denied her hostile feelings, finding, as she put it, "Some good in everyone."

Louise later married a weak, somewhat inadequate man, and spent her life taking care of him and their four children. She worked very hard at this role. As one of the children pointed out, "When Bobby broke his leg, she carried him to school on her back." Indeed, she carried the whole family on her back in a figurative sense, frequently supporting the family with her wages, while at the same time acting as nurse, mother and housekeeper.

After fifteen years of marriage, Louise's husband died. But she successfully raised the children, all four of whom went into fields demanding high intellectual activity. In spite of economic pressures, she led a happy life until the youngest child grew up and went to work. She went to live with this son. His job took him from town to town for assignments lasting from one to three years, and she went with him, cooking and keeping house. Finally, though, it became clear to her that her son no longer needed her and would be happier without her.

Louise then entered into a period of confusion and dismay. She tried various occupations and hobbies but could not really arouse her interest in any of them. For a time she did very little at all. She became quieter and more relaxed than the children had ever seen her. They thought the change was "wonderful." But in actuality Louise had lost her role, the central relationship around which she had built her life. She was unable to find any new outlet for her emotions. What she had found was not peace, as her children thought, but despair. And about a year after she stopped keeping house for her youngest son, her breast cancer developed.

For the individual who has lost a central relationship, a role that gave meaning to his or her life, there is thus a double blockage. On the one hand, like Louise and Arthur, the person is deprived of the outlet for the emotions that had caused life to be worthwhile. Yet there is also an inability to express the resentment or hostility that this loss creates. Both kinds of blockage feed the despair of the individual, creating the kind of emotional climate in which resistance to cancer appears to be lowered.

The Emotional Life History of Cancer Patients

Why, it may be asked, doesn't the individual deprived of his *raison d'être,* seek out new possibilities, new relationships?

Many of my patients had in fact tried to do this. Arthur devoted more time to his family and tried to interest himself in a variety of volunteer organizations. Louise made efforts to find an occupation that would give her the satisfaction that raising and caring for her children had provided. Catherine, prevented from pursuing her musical studies in the environment she wished, got married.

Yet in each case, these efforts failed. The reasons for their failure, and for the growing despair that each of these people faced, appear to be strongly connected with the loss that each suffered in childhood. No matter how long their relationship—to a person, a group, a role, a talent that gave them a sense of purpose—had lasted, whether it was one year or forty years, all the old doubts of their childhood came flooding back. The relationship had made it possible for them to forget their feelings of self-contempt, to repress their sense that there was something wrong with them, something that made them unacceptable to others. But once the relationship ended, it was as though it had been erased—as though the satisfactions that it had offered meant nothing.

These individuals did not say to themselves, "Well, I was happy for that time, life was meaningful, and if I could feel that way once I can do so again." Indeed, they

61

felt the opposite. The relationship that had sustained them seemed a lucky chance, a good thing that had happened *to* them, rather than a good thing that they had *caused* to happen. They took no credit for their own satisfaction. The happiness they had felt did not persuade them that they did indeed deserve to be happy. Instead, they saw the end of the relationship as a disaster that they had always half-expected. They had been waiting for it to end, waiting for rejection. It was, they felt, their destiny to be rejected. And when it happened, they said to themselves, "Yes, I always knew it was too good to be true."

This thought was not, in most cases, given such explicit expression, at least until they entered therapy. But it gives the gist of what they felt to be true. Like Sisyphus, again, they had always been certain that they would never reach the top of the mountain, that sooner or later the rock would roll back to the bottom. The end of their special relationship simply proved to them that they had been right.

From a superficial point of view, all managed to "adjust" to the blow. They continued to function. They went about their daily business. But the "color," the zest, the meaning went out of their lives. They no longer seemed attached to life. In the words of T.S. Eliot, they saw their lives as being empty:

Shape without form, shade without colour
Paralyzed force, gesture without motion. . .

They made the gesture, they continued to carry out the day-to-day tasks of life, but the gesture was without a sense of forward motion. They had no hope of the future, and no conviction that the gesture itself held any meaning.

To those around them, even people close to them, they seemed to be coping perfectly well. In some cases, as with Louise's children, other people thought them to be more content, more at peace than they had ever been. But in fact, it was the false peace of despair that they felt. They were simply waiting to die. For that seemed to them the only way out. They were ready for death. In one very real sense, they had already died. One patient said to me, "Last time I hoped, and look what happened. As soon as my defenses were down, of course I was left alone again. I'll never hope again. It's too much. It's better to stay in a shell."

And there they stayed, waiting without hope for death to release them. Within six months to eight years, among my patients, the terminal cancer appeared.

This basic emotional life history was found to prevail in 76% of all the cancer patients I studied, including those for whom I had only test protocols available, or with whom I had only conducted short interviews. Among the non-cancer control patients, this emotional pattern was found among only 10%. Of the cancer patients who came to me for intensive psychotherapy, 66 out of the 71 conformed to this pattern. The fact that a higher percentage (over 95%) was found among the psychotherapy patients than held true for the entire group studied is of particular interest. It may be that this was part of the self-selection process that brought these patients into psychotherapy. It should also be remembered that all of the patients in therapy were given no medical hope of cure or even of survival beyond a period of a few months: either their tumors were inoperable or had spread beyond control. This was not necessarily the case with the patients studied by means of the test protocols or the short interviews. Thus there are indications that the degree of emotional estrangement from life on the part of an individual may affect the severity and virulence of the cancer itself. This is a subject I will be returning to in a subsequent chapter.

The basic emotional pattern of the cancer patient appears, on the basis of my observations, to have three major parts. The first part involves a childhood or adolescence marked by feelings of isolation. There is a sense that intense and meaningful relationships are dangerous and bring pain and rejection. The second part of the pattern is centered upon the period during which a meaningful relationship is discovered, allowing the individual to enjoy a sense of acceptance by others (at least in one particular role) and to find a meaning to his life. The third aspect of the pattern comes to the fore when the loss of that central relationship occurs. Now there is a sense of utter despair, connected to but going beyond the childhood sense of isolation. In this third phase, the conviction that life holds no more hope becomes paramount. And sometime after the onset of the third phase, the first symptoms of cancer are noted.

Linking these three phases together is a particular perception of the universe. The way in which the cancer patient typically views the way his world works —and has always viewed his world, from childhood on —is distinctive. His outlook is basically a mechanistic one: the "cold, clockmaker's universe" described by the 17th-century French philosopher and mathematician Descartes. But Descartes, although he could well be called the father of "modern" thought, was comforted in his vision of a mechanistic world by his belief in a warm and loving presence of God. That presence is absent for the typical cancer patient. Rather, the cancer patient has a sense of *Moira,* a weaving of fate that seems to each individual to apply to himself alone.

Perceiving the cosmos as uncaring and unconcerned, the typical cancer victim does not conceive of any meaning beyond the human being and his particular relationships. Yet, at the same time, the individual has the feeling that he has been singled out by fate. No matter what he does, how hard he tries, the course of his life is seen as predetermined, joyless and doomed. There seems to be little paranoid element in this concept, however. Indeed, it rests in that almost subliminal level of feeling where most of us in the 20th-century hold our assumptions about the nature of the universe. Working with these patients, it seemed to me that this concept of personal doom had been fundamental to their belief since childhood. Even in the best moments of their lives the sense of a predetermined fate remained in the background, a distant but still ominous drum roll.

The cancer patient's concept of the universe can perhaps be made still clearer by making use of the ideas of the Swiss psychiatrist Ludwig·Binswanger, who conceives of the individual as living in three worlds. First there is the *umwelt:* the environment and the world of things. The world of others is called the *mitwelt*. Finally, the *gegenwelt* is the self, the inner world. Among my patients the *umwelt* seemed to be quite unimportant. Even those people who were striving for material success, and might be expected to place considerable emphasis on the world of things, did not do so. They were not interested in the acquisition of money and things for the sake of having them. Rather their hard work, their material striving, was a desperate attempt to find satisfaction in life through the medium of objects, even though they "knew" (both consciously and on deeper levels) that such objects could not satisfy their hunger. For most of my patients, their work was a method by which they might try to reach out and communicate with others— much as a chess game may be used as a social device to establish a relationship with an opponent.

The *mitwelt,* or world of others, seemed to my patients to be determined on the basis of an either/or principle. In accordance with the personality factors discussed in previous chapters, they felt they must either conform or be rejected, and were unable to conceive of any middle path. They believed that if they wished to be loved, and to be given the same acceptance that they understood other people to receive, it would be necessary for them to conform to certain demands of thought, feeling and behavior. If they did not or could not conform, it seemed to them, they would be rejected, would be outsiders cast into cold loneliness. To be loved, they must be untrue to themselves. And this either/or view of the possibilities of relationship with others was completely inflexible. It seemed incomprehensible to them that it could be possible to modify *some* unimportant parts of their behavior, and thus be accepted by others even while retaining their own thoughts and feelings.

Many of these individuals were terribly alert to each new person that entered their environment. Would the new person, as expected, reject them? One patient told me, "My radar is always out 50 miles." But even as my patients had always feared rejection, they had at the same time courted it. They created test after test for any potential friend, lover or spouse. If the new person failed one test, it was enough to convince the patient that his or her fears were indeed legitimate: he or she was, as expected, unlovable. If a test was passed, a new one was always devised. One test after another followed until, at last, the predicted failure to respond occurred. As Alma put it: "It's no wonder no man ever loved me. They were all too tired after climbing over all that barbed wire to get to me."

This either/or, "all or none" perspective was also applied to the self, or *gegenwelt*. These individuals could break, but they could not bend. "Here I stand," they

67

seem to say. "I can do nothing else." They have a dim perception of what they need in order to be themselves, to express themselves fully as human beings. But to do so, to be creative in this special way that would fulfill their unique selves, will only bring complete rejection, closing the channel to others once again, brutally—they are convinced of it. Because the closing of that channel is always accompanied by overwhelming anguish, their emotional reactions to others are often so defensive that they tend to provoke the feared rejection. Or that rejection may be perceived where it does not exist.

Virginia, while believing that no man could ever fully love her, met a married man with whom she wanted to have an affair. The man was much in love with her, but felt that adultery was wrong for both of them, that it would destroy their feelings for one another. He urged that they should each divorce their spouses and marry one another. But this response—one that in most relationships would be the ultimate proof of the man's love —was taken by Virginia as a rejection. She saw it not as evidence of love, but as one more example of the lack of love that had always been her fate.

The "desired self" of these patients, the essence of what they wanted to be as human beings, was of a nature that made it impossible of achievement. Almost without exception, they made "gigantic claims" (as Karen Horney has termed them) against themselves. The standards they set for themselves were beyond human fulfillment. But these ideals were at the same time often very vague, and expressed far more in terms of "don'ts" than dos." Thus, even if by some miracle the patient might reach his goal, he probably would not recognize the fact.

When, in the course of therapy, these tremendous claims against the self were verbalized, the patients were generally able to see their ridiculous nature and to laugh at them—but only very slowly were they able to abandon them. "If I can realize these ambitions," they appeared to be saying, "then others *must* accept and love me. Then I can really be a part of this world, bound to it by the response of others."

But with standards of such magnitude, no degree of actual success was ever seen as being close enough to the ideal. No matter what was achieved, it never seemed to make any real difference. Recognition and respect from others, even when it was very considerable and came in an area where it was particularly desired, seemed hollow and unconvincing. Alma, for example, had been offered the perfect job for her rare combination of talents. In spite of a great need by the organization that hired her, the position had remained open for 5 years because they had not been able to find a person with the varied abilities required. Alma did an outstanding job in the position, but it in no way increased her self-respect or self-confidence.

Virginia was a stunningly lovely woman, but she did not conceive of herself as attractive to men. She desperately needed masculine response, and, in fact, many men of high caliber were attracted to her. She was courted, had several affairs and many proposals, but still she could not change her claim that she was unattractive to men. Even when she understood how often an attraction had been demonstrated, how high her "score" was, it made no difference. In a humorous vein, I suggested possible actions that *would* convince her of her own appeal: men shooting themselves by the thousands for love of her, the Foreign Legion overrun by enlistees trying to forget her, first prize in the "Miss Universe" contest followed by abandonment of future competitions because no one could hope to measure up to her. She laughed, and said, "I guess you're getting close to what I have in mind, but you still have a way to go." She saw the absurdity of her claim as to what she "should be," but could not relinquish it. At the same time, of course, she also felt that she should be a quiet housewife and mother, faithful and loving to her husband, always available to her children, a perfect daughter who gave her mother every attention, not to mention a scientist who "did things for the world like Madame Curie."

Here again, the reader may feel a certain impatience with Virginia, and with people like her. How absurd to be so demanding of oneself! But for all the absurdity of Virginia's feelings about herself and the world, they are *real* feelings, deeply held. So deeply held, in fact, that they created in her an unbearable anguish. So deeply held, in fact, that they appear to have predisposed her to the onslaught of cancer. It is both a glory and a tragedy of the human mind and spirit that what we "feel" to be true about ourselves, no matter how farfetched, often becomes actualized. The person who is convinced that success will come often succeeds far beyond what his or her native abilities might suggest. The person who is convinced that failure is inevitable, often fails in spite of a high degree of actual ability. The terminal cancer patient almost always expects failure and rejection. When a central relationship founders, the patient is not surprised—that is what has always been feared and anticipated. The cancer itself, when it appears, is viewed in the same way.

My own understanding of the personality of the cancer patient has been corroborated by others. Dr. Gotthard Booth, a New York psychiatrist, noted a similar pattern among 125 of his cancer patients. Many of them, he found, had been "dominated since childhood by the feeling that their opportunities for satisfaction are very limited and that they would succeed only with great effort in creating a meaningful existence for themselves. A severe loss, particularly in the years of declining vitality, is therefore experienced as irretrievable."

From my own studies, I would say that the sense of irretrievable loss can come at any age. The personality of the cancer patient is such that a severe loss of relationship at any point in life brings on despair. There is, of course, a seeming contradiction here. The cancer patient has more emotion than he or she is able to express —yet finds it impossible to draw upon this emotion in defense of the self. Since the self is found wanting, incapable of achieving the impossible goals that have been set, the emotional needs of the patient cannot be met.

You Can Fight for Your Life

The emotional force, like an inland pool that has neither fresh inlets nor outward flow, stagnates and becomes a kind of bog in which only the organisms of decay can find a home. Yet, just as it is possible to restore to environmental health a stagnant pool, by digging a trench that will connect it with living streams in the surrounding area, so too can the channel to the outer world be opened again for the cancer patient. Before discussing how this channel can be re-opened, however, there is more to learn about the emotional life history of the cancer patient.

Stress and Susceptibility 5

From my clinical study of cancer patients, as well as control patients, a definite picture had emerged during the first five years of my research. This picture, both in its overall outlines and in its details, indicated that there was a structure of personality and a structure of emotional life history that was typical for cancer patients—and atypical for the controls. Cancer patients—particularly those whose malignancy was regarded as terminal and beyond medical help—seemed to be a particular kind of people.

Yet this picture remained hypothetical. Provocative,

stimulating and useful though the results of my study had proved to be, it remained necessary to test the hypothesis by other methods in order to ascertain its scientific validity. The understanding of the personality of the cancer patient that I had gradually developed had made it possible for me to help a number of my patients to find new hope for themselves, to change their view of the world and achieve a greater sense of satisfaction during the time left to them than they had ever experienced. For a few, the restoration of hope had been accompanied by a remission of the cancer itself. The rebirth of hope in these patients—whose cases I will present in detail later on—was strong evidence that my hypothesis was correct. But it was not "objective" evidence of the kind required in constructing a scientific proof.

In experimental psychology and most other sciences, a widely used method for testing hypotheses is to predict the data that should result from other modes of research. Thus a heart specialist might predict that men who smoke and drink fairly heavily will be more likely to suffer coronary attacks. To test this hypothesis two groups of volunteers—one group composed of men who did smoke and drink, the other of men who did not—would be intensively studied at the outset and then regularly rechecked over a period of perhaps ten years. Because of the long latency period associated with cancer, it is difficult to set up a statistically valid research project of this type. However, there is a second approach that offers more immediate results. This method involves the prediction of relative cancer mortality rates for different groups, with the prediction to be tested against data already gathered by other researchers. For instance, I had found that the loss of a central relationship generally preceded the development of a fatal malignancy. If this observation were correct, then cancer mortality rates among women, for instance, ought to reflect the likelihood that they had lost such a central relationship. In fact, it ought to vary according to the marital status of the women.

Thus the marital group with the highest cancer mortality rate should be the "widowed." Among this group, the loss of a spouse due to illness or accident should most frequently have meant the loss of an intense relationship. The next highest cancer mortality rate should be among the "divorced." The mortality rate for divorced women would be lower than for widows in that fewer of the divorced women would have been likely to make their marriages the major focus of their emotional energies. Yet the rate for divorced women would be higher than for the "married." That is, a larger percentage of divorced individuals would have had a crucial relationship formed and lost than would be the case among either the "married" or "single" groups.

The rate would be higher for the "married" group than the "single," according to similar reasoning. Among married individuals, the emotional bond may have been broken, even though the couple remained legally bound because of religion, custom, or economic pressures. The lowest cancer mortality rate should be found among the "single" group, because these individuals would have least often established and lost a central relationship in the marital area.

Simply stated, the prediction was that the cancer rates of women should be related to their marital status. Of the four marital classes, the cancer mortality rates should be highest among the widowed, then among the divorced, then among the married, and least among the single.

This prediction was indeed borne out by statistics gathered from several sources. R. A. Herring, for example, reported on the mortality rate for women in the United States during the 1929-31 period. He used the data of the Bureau of the Census, and took his figures directly from birth certificates. His analysis is shown in Table I.

TABLE I

Cancer Mortality Rates Per 100,000 Living Population
of United States 1929–31, Females Only

	Breast	Uterus	Ovary, Fallopian Tubes	Vulva and Vagina	All Other Sites	Total
Single	15.0	9.0	3.3	.5	33.4	61.2
Married	24.5	35.0	4.7	.8	11.8	137.7
Divorced	29.3	57.2	6.0	1.5	81.8	175.8
Widowed	74.4	94.4	9.6	4.3	344.4	527.1

It may be objected that any disease which is more common among older people would show the same type of relationship to marital status. But this is not the case, according to available statistics. The two disorders whose age-grading appears to be most clearly parallel to cancer are heart disease and diabetes. No statistics relating to marital status are available for heart disease. But a study on the death rate in England and Wales for diabetes during 1931-32, shows that the relationship between cancer and marital status that can be seen in Table I does not exist where diabetes is concerned. In fact, as shown in Table II, the death rate from diabetes was generally higher for married women than widows, even at more advanced ages. This fact reinforces the idea that there is a special relationship between marital status and cancer, regardless of the age factors involved.

TABLE II

Death Rate Per Million from Diabetes
England and Wales 1931–32, Females Only

AGE	30	35	40	45	50	55	60	65	70	75
Married	48	59	68	88	183	305	491	722	751	723
Widowed	41	42	41	111	178	321	502	627	737	646

An English researcher, S. Peller, made a careful analysis of the cancer data published by the British government for 1932, and found that "in comparing the death rates for single women and widows, the latter in all age groups are significantly higher." The rates were also higher, he found, for the widowed than for the married

77

at all age levels. Peller summed up one part of his research by saying:

> . . . the less satisfactory the marital status, the earlier the patient manifests cancer and dies from it . . . . the circumstances attendant upon the husband's death are apt to increase the mortality from both uterine and breast cancer.

A number of other studies showed similar results. I could find no study that contradicted my prediction that mortality rates would vary according to marital status. This material has been published elsewhere (see Bibliography), and is thus available to the medical community. It seems unnecessary, therefore, to burden the general reader with additional statistical data on this point. The results were strikingly clear: the prediction that cancer deaths would be most common for widows and least common for single women was borne out by the existing studies.

On the basis of my general hypothesis, it was also possible to make other predictions that could be tested against data gathered by other researchers. In discussing the "married" group in previous pages, I noted that in many situations a marriage might remain legally intact even though it has deteriorated from a psychological viewpoint. Under such circumstances, the central relationship may have been lost even though the couple remains together. This was a major consideration in predicting that the mortality rate would be higher for the married group than for the single. But there is a further point that can be made about the married group.

Within the married group itself are two subgroups: the "married with children" and the "married without children." Suppose that a couple is psychologically estranged, even though they remain together. A central relationship has been lost. Then let us ask ourselves which couple is most likely, as individuals, to have found a successful substitute relationship, one that is sufficiently sustaining as to provide the emotional outlet crucial to a sense of hope and of the value of life. Clearly the married couple with children is more likely to have found a valid new relationship, involving those children. Even though the relationship between the husband and wife may have lost its original meaning and strength, each of them has the possibility of funneling his or her emotional needs into a substitute relationship with the children.

For this prediction to have meaning, it is necessary for the same type of variation to hold for the males and females involved. If only the females show the predicted mortality variation by marital status, it might be assumed that the variation is due to hormonal factors. But if the males show a similar variation, then the explanation must lie elsewhere than in hormonal factors, giving further weight to the emotional element under consideration here.

Thus, we can make the prediction that among both men and women, the cancer mortality rate will be higher for married individuals without children than for those who do have children. This prediction is, indeed, borne out by a statistical report on the total population of Australia for the years 1919-23. H. Dorn demonstrated that the mortality rate was lower for those with children, and that this factor held true for both males and females.

TABLE III

Cancer Mortality Rates, Total Population of Australia

	MARRIED MALES WITH CHILDREN	SINGLE MALES	MARRIED MALES WITHOUT CHILDREN
1919–23	163	168	182

(Dorn reports that the figures for 1921-31 and for 1931–35 are in "substantial agreement" with the figures presented.)

	MARRIED FEMALES WITH CHILDREN	SINGLE FEMALES	MARRIED FEMALES WITHOUT CHILDREN
1919–23	163	179	183
1931–35	152	166	193

The reader may be puzzled by the figures for single males and single females above, since they are higher

80

than for the married with children groups. These statistics do not, as it might seem, contradict my earlier prediction that mortality rates would be higher for the married than the single. In making that previous prediction, no distinction was made between married individuals with children and those without. If the figures for those with children and those without in the above table are averaged together, the rate for this over-all "married" group is indeed higher. It was exactly because I expected such a variation when the married group was subdivided that I looked for further evidence.

It should by now be clear to the reader that any situation that tends to disrupt the formation of strong, meaningful relationships can be predicted to result in higher cancer mortality rates. For instance, we know from various studies that second generation Americans as a group show many more indications of social disruption than do either first or third generation Americans. The first generation immigrants still have the mores and viewpoints of their country of origin to bind them together. The third generation citizens have acquired the orientations of their new culture. The second generation group, however, caught between the viewpoint of their parents and the viewpoints of the larger society, tends to be the least well adjusted and the least cohesive of the three generations. This second generation may thus be assumed to have a larger percentage of lost relationships. Therefore, we would predict that the second generation group would have higher cancer mortality rates than either the first or third generation group.

A study by Bigelow and Lombard presents the data relevant to this prediction, as shown in **Table IV.**

TABLE IV

Age and Sex Corrected Cancer Mortality Rates, Massachusetts, 1928

	NATIVE BORN OF NATIVE PARENTS	FOREIGN BORN	NATIVE BORN OF FOREIGN PARENTS
Males	74.8±3.1*	146±4.3	235.0±9.8
Females	129.2±4.0	179±4.8	281.0±9.8

* ± refers to probable error

The much higher death rate among the second generation shown in this table is striking evidence of the validity of this prediction—and of the basic hypothesis that lost relationships contribute importantly to the development of cancer.

Moving into a still broader arena, let us consider what happens to relationships in wartime. A number of sociologists and psychologists have pointed out that when a country is at war, group cohesiveness increases as common goals and efforts bind people together more tightly. This is only true, of course, where the country as a whole is deeply involved in the war over a fairly long period of time. The end of a war, however, is likely to produce the opposite effect. There are changes in the economy, post-war fantasies fail to materialize, the common enemy no longer exists, the quest for victory is past—and all these factors can produce bitterness, disappointment, and loss of group solidarity.

We would expect that these changes would be reflected in the inter-personal relationships formed by individuals, and we might therefore predict that cancer rates would decrease during wartime and increase in the post-war years in countries which were wholeheartedly engaged in war. Furthermore, we would expect that if we could find a country which was markedly disorganized by war, with sharply different opinions of great emotional strength held by different members of the population, then this would tend to disrupt relationships—and we might predict an abnormally high cancer rate.

In fact, cancer mortality rates in both Denmark and England showed a significant decrease during World War I, and a temporary significant rise after the armistice. During the years 1942–45, there was an "inexplicable" temporary rise in cancer mortality rates in Ireland. Ireland was a country in which very strong, differing emotional responses occurred during World War II. On the one hand, there was a revulsion for the nature of the Nazi movement. But at the same time, the traditional Irish dislike and distrust of England continued to be felt, accompanied by ambivalence due to the fact that many young Irishmen joined the British army. Thus the rise in cancer mortality rates is not inexplicable according to my hypothesis; quite the contrary, it is exactly what would be expected.

I also carried out other objective tests. Several of these involved statistical analysis of a nature too complex to be fully reported here. But a general statement of the kinds of predictions involved can be made. I predicted, for instance, that differences in cancer mortality rates should be found among individuals suffering from different sub-types of schizophrenia. It was predicted that paranoid schizophrenics, because they were most likely to have had strong relationships prior to the onset of their psychosis, would have abnormally high cancer mortality rates. Other types of schizophrenic—the hebephrenic, catatonic and simple—who tended to make only weak relationships prior to the onset of their psychosis were predicted to have abnormally low rates. These predictions were corroborated by three separate studies of cancer rates among institutionalized mental patients.

Drawing upon another aspect of my over-all hypothesis, the concept that the cancer patient had an orientation in childhood that emotional relationships were dangerous, another set of statistical tests were made. This work was done in collaboration with Marvin Reznikoff, Ph.D., and was first published jointly with him. Dr. Reznikoff had previously published a study showing that a statistically significant higher number of his cancer patients had had a brother or sister die in childhood than was the case with cancer-free individuals whom he used as a control. Using the information already amassed by Dr. Reznikoff, as well as a Danish study by O. Jacobsen, further testing was done. We believed that cancer patients were likely to have had less time as "the baby" of the family, due to the birth of another child, and thus less time to fill their dependency needs in the ideal family situation. We found that individuals with cancer do tend to have a shorter period of being the youngest child than do their cancer-free brothers and sisters.

This study seemed to be particularly important. Not only did it appear to confirm the general hypothesis that cancer patients, early in life, developed the feeling that emotional relationships were dangerous, it also provided new information as to why they might feel that way. Among the more than fifty patients I had treated in intensive psychotherapy, many had suffered some acute loss as a child, the death of a parent or sibling, or separation from one or both parents in either a physical or emotional way. This kind of loss was, as we have previously noted, far more common for the cancer patients than for my patients without cancer. Nevertheless, it did not apply to all my cancer patients. What had caused them to develop the feelings that emotional relationships were dangerous? Now, there was the beginning of an answer to that question. Clearly, the birth of a sibling could cause the parents to transfer their attention to this new member of the family; and if the older child had not had sufficient time to fill his dependency needs, the loss of his parents' undivided attention could be traumatic enough to make him feel that relationships in general were dangerous and anxiety-provoking.

You Can Fight for Your Life

Since I concluded my own testing, other researchers have made similar findings in regard to several aspects of the personality of the cancer patient as I came to understand it in the course of my own research. For instance, Dr. Arthur H. Schmale and Dr. Howard Iker of the University of Rochester found their cancer patients to be self-contained, rigid and often withdrawn. They were undemonstrative, being neither openly affectionate nor openly angry. These two physicians found this pattern so compelling that they attempted to predict the presence or absence of cancer, on the basis of psychiatric interviews alone, for a group of 69 women who had entered the hospital for a cervical biopsy. Their degree of accuracy in making these predictions was 72.5%.

Dr. Claus Bahnson, of the Eastern Pennsylvania Psychiatric Institute compared three different groups: cancer patients, patients with other illnesses, and a group of healthy individuals. Unlike the other two groups, the cancer patients had a history of cold and unsatisfying relationships with their parents. "People with this kind of background," Dr. Bahnson states, "are more vulnerable to the effects of loss in later life, because they have difficulty maintaining close relationships and lack an outlet for intensified emotional charges."

The lack of an outlet for intensified emotional charges seems to me particularly important. Among the patients whom I treated in intensive psychotherapy (as well as those with whom I conducted short interviews) I was struck by a recurring impression that these people had a strong basic quality of "elan vital." The vital force seemed somehow stronger in them than in the controls. Even when its lustre was dimmed by despair, these individuals seemed to have a special "spark," a strong potential for being alive.

It is difficult to define the source of this very strong impression. Conceivably, it could have been related to the "bottled up" quality of their lives, the presence of more emotional energy than they had ways of expressing it. All of them had needs to be creative and to relate to others in more ways than they felt were available to them. But beyond this, it seemed as though they simply had more inner "fire" than would be found in a normal cross-section of the population. This impression was so strong and consistent that I often found myself speculating whether cancer might not be a selective disease that is more likely to appear in those with the highest level of emotional force, especially if their lives did not allow for the full venting of that force.

In recent years, a number of researchers have taken particular note of the apparent suppression of emotion among the patients they have studied. I have already mentioned the work of Dr. David Kissen of Glasgow, who found that cancer patients showed a "poor outlet for emotional discharge," and were less able to express their feelings. A psychiatrist at Memorial Sloan-Kettering Cancer Center in New York, Dr. Rene Mastrovito, studied a group of women with cancer of the reproductive tract. He found these patients to have a high degree of "emotional self-control, idealism and sense of responsibility."

Emotional self-control. Idealism. Responsibility. We are taught that all of these qualities are virtues, and there is no doubt that they are, when they appear in the proper context. But even a virtue can be carried to extremes. If responsibility and self-control are rigidly maintained at the expense of the expression of genuine feelings, a part of the self is denied. When tensions are not released, when anger is repressed, it can begin to feed upon itself. We know that this happens in the development of ulcers. Can we deny the possibility that it also occurs in the development of cancers?

One must be responsible for and to others, certainly. But one must also be responsible to and for one's self. The juvenile delinquent, refusing to accept his responsibility toward others, expresses his anger in outward anti-social acts. But may not the person whose sense of responsibility toward others obliterates his sense of responsibility to himself take out his anger upon himself? In his book *How Will You Feel Tomorrow*, Dr. Samuel Silverman of the Harvard Medical School notes that when anger, grief or severe worry have no outlet, they eventually affect the body. "If there is a latent tendency to develop a cancerous growth," he writes, "a failure to express emotional feelings will hit the body in a vulnerable spot."

At present, cancer researchers generally believe that cancer cells are almost continuously present in all of us but that our "cancer immune system" seeks out and destroys these aberrant cells, under normal circumstances, thus preventing their growth or spread. The question remains as to what constitutes the abnormal circumstances that may prevent the immune system from doing its job. What physical mechanism of the body is sufficiently influenced by psychological factors to provide a link between the emotions and the breakdown of the cancer immune system?

Current research points to the endocrine system and the hormones it produces. We know that certain hormones affect the growth and spread of cancer. We also know that psychological factors can alter the body's hormonal balance. Vernon Riley has shown that environmental stress can shorten the period it takes for mammary tumors to develop in mice. Dr. John W. Mason of the Walter Reed Institute of Research has demonstrated that stress produces a wide variety of hormonal changes in rhesus monkeys, and that certain kinds of stress produce particular hormonal changes.

Much further research needs to be done before this linkage can be pinpointed. Yet my own work with terminal cancer patients convinces me that such work is moving in the right direction. Certainly my patients were affected by a remarkably consistent pattern of stress. Their personalities and life histories put them under particular kinds of stress generally not found in my non-cancer patients. When that stress was relieved, the growth of their cancers was often affected dramatically. Usually, these changes took place over a period of months or years. John's brain tumor, for instance, gradually decreased over a period of three years. But sometimes changes could be noted in the course of a few hours.

One of my patients, a 32-year-old woman, had visible nodes in the neck and shoulder region, a symptom of Hodgkin's disease. When she began therapy with me, a curious recurrent pattern showed itself. The evening before a therapy session, the nodes tended to increase in size, and to decease on the evening following the session. A very real change in the size of the swelling could be observed by herself and her family in the course of a few hours. This phenomenon occurred in connection with about half her therapy sessions, and then disappeared after the first three months of therapy.

Another case, reported to me by Dr. Albert Kean, a radiologist with exceptionally broad experience in the field of Hodgkin's disease, involved a 19-year-old woman who was not in psychotherapy. Her only symptoms were small scattered nodes on the neck; Kean decided to keep her under weekly observation. For three months no changes were observed. Then, on a weekly visit, the girl came in with one side of her neck extremely distended. The existing nodes had markedly increased in size and new ones had appeared. Kean questioned her as to whether anything unusual had happened in the previous week. The young woman told him that she had informed her fiancé that she had Hodgkin's disease. He very much wanted children, and feeling that she couldn't have any, he broke off the engagement. Shortly afterwards, her neck began to swell.

In view of this unusual situation, Kean asked the fiancé to come in to see him, and discussed the course of the young woman's disease and its prognosis. The man, having recovered from the shock of the news, realized that the illness did not really matter to him and that he did in fact want to marry the girl. He told her so, and within three days the nodes returned to the size that they had been before the engagement was broken. No radiation or other therapy had been used during that three-day interval.

Such connections between the emotions and bodily reactions are, of course, notoriously difficult to study in traditional scientific ways. Yet human beings have always been aware of their importance. Galen, the Greek physician of the second century A.D., attributed cancer to a melancholy disposition. Approaching the question from the same direction, medieval physicians attempted to explain personality according to the presence or lack of such supposed bodily constitutents as "bile" and "phlegm"—a primitive attempt to define the hormonal activities uncovered by modern medical science. As our knowledge of bodily processes has increased over the centuries, emotional factors have sometimes been pushed into the background. But the theme is recurrent. A century ago, Sir James Paget, one of the outstanding figures in this field, wrote this about cancer: "The cases are so frequent in which deep anxiety,

91

deferred hope and disappointment are quickly followed by the growth and increase of cancer that we can hardly doubt that mental depression is a weighty additive to the other influences favoring the development of the cancerous constitution." Such ideas went into eclipse again during the first half of our own century, as purely physical modes of treatment were improved in leap after forward leap. Thus my own initial research was met with great skepticism among the medical community. But now, as it becomes increasingly clear that physical explanations—environment, viral, or genetic —do not provide the whole answer, more and more physicians and psychologists are looking for additional information in regard to the influence of stress, personality and the emotions.

Among my own patients, I found that there seemed to be a general correspondence between the rate at which a malignancy developed and the length of time that had elapsed since that individual had lost his sense of life's meaning as embodied in a central relationship. The shorter the period, the more rapid was the development of the cancer. Thus patients in whom a tumor was diagnosed shortly after the loss of their central relationship (six months to a year) tended to have rapid tumor development. Those for whom this period was longer (two years to eight years) tended to have a moderate or slow tumor development. Obviously, those with a slow development have a better chance at survival.

Other researchers have made similar observations.

Dr. Bruno Klopfer was able to predict with nearly 80% accuracy which patients had slow-growing cancers, and which fast-growing, on the basis of personality tests alone. "The only explanation that makes sense to me," he said, "is a symbiotic relationship between the patient and his cancer. If a good deal of the vital energy the patient has at his disposal is used up in the defense of a insecure ego, then the organism seems not to have the vital energy to fight the cancer off . . . If, however, a minimum of vital energy is consumed in ego defensiveness, then the cancer has a hard time making headway."

My own patients were nearly all regarded, medically speaking, as beyond help; their cancers were terminal. Some, however, did have more resources than others with which to fight for their lives. Those who were most completely in despair, who most thoroughly lost their sense of life's meaning, had the least resources.

To fight for your life, you must have the resources of self-acceptance and self-approval. It was my job as a psychotherapist to help my patients regain those resources, so that they would be able to fight. I could not cure cancer. But I could help my patients to care enough once more—for themselves and for what their lives might be—so that they themselves could fight against the malignancy with the whole of their new-found emotional strength.

During the first few years of my research I had established to my own satisfaction that there was indeed a connection between personality and cancer. Now, I

93

Psychotherapy and the Cancer Patient 6

The daughter of one of my patients wrote to me after her mother's death: ". . . I know that every day she grew in courage and understanding and was learning to fight the fears that surrounded her. With a woman like Mother—I suppose with any human being—an illness such as hers could have been the final fear to entirely hem her in and shut her off from human contact. But I do think that through her work with you, she somehow managed to win through her illness to a greater understanding, not only of herself but of other people too. So please don't feel that your work was in vain.

I don't believe that anything like that ever goes into a vacuum. Somehow it perpetuates itself. My father and I are changed because of the change in Mother, and I think it influenced her friends who visited her. Because of you, Mother's last months were filled with hope and thoughts of the future, to her very last hours."

I quote these words not as a matter of self-congratulation, but because they encapsulate so many of the difficulties and the potentials of psychotherapy with terminally ill patients. The ultimate potential of such therapy, of course, is to help effect a "cure" or a remission of the cancer itself. In a few cases, as we shall see, that goal was achieved. But the therapist must avoid raising false hopes. Therapy with a terminally ill patient should concentrate on the expansion, growth and freeing of the self rather than upon physical recovery. The therapist needs to have the courage to say, in effect, "We do not know what the outcome will be, but we will do our best. The psychological work you and I do here can only be beneficial in effect. It may help. It will help you find life more worth fighting for, and the harder one fights, the better chance one has in anything. But there are no promises or guarantees. I can no more make them than the universe makes them." Generally, the patient will find this approach acceptable. As Laurens White has pointed out, "Our patients do not ask us to cure them. They ask us to care for them and to take care of them."

With cancer patients, I found that the mere fact of my actually *caring* was of great value. To the patient, the fact of someone's believing in him enough to really work at helping him toward greater self-understanding and inner growth in the midst of catastrophe has a very positive impact. The patient is all too aware that he most likely will not be able to "repay" the therapist by a long future period of adequate functioning. Traditional psychotherapy is future-oriented. It is a common basic assumption of such psychotherapy that the psychotherapist works with a patient to increase the value of his long-term productivity and his long-term relationships with others, and, perhaps, to better his adjustment to the environment. Clearly, these are not valid goals for the patient with a fatal illness.

But if I could not work on the basis of such assumptions, what approach could or should I take? The philosopher Martin Heidegger provides a clue in his suggestion that the age of a man should be reckoned not only in terms of how long he has lived, but also of how long he has yet to live. Within this frame of reference, what the person IS and DOES during the remainder of his life span is of major importance; that is, what his life encompasses in feeling and understanding rather than how long it lasts in a purely chronological sense. In "crisis therapy"—which is the term I use to describe the therapeutic approaches and techniques I developed for use with terminal cancer patients—life can be seen more validly as an extension in values than as an extension in time. "The longest necessary life is until a man is wise," wrote Seneca. If a person has one hour to live and for the first time fully discovers himself and his life in that hour, is not this a valid and important growth?

Thus, when I began to work with cancer patients, I sought to reawaken the inner life of the individual, and to liberate those forces which can enable the person to experience as completely as possible both himself and the meaning of his life and death. If we believe in the value of the individual and the sacred character of human life, our concern does not stop as death approaches. The responsibility of the therapist is not limited to certain stages of development. A patient of mine with a wide-spread abdominal cancer said to his 21-year-old daughter, "Death is nothing. It is inevitable. Everyone has to die. What matters is *how* you live and die. That's what Larry and I are talking about: *Style!*" This statement was made after thirty hours of psychotherapy and was evidence that we had come a long way. Such words could be spoken only by a person who has begun to come to terms with the facts of his life and his death.

Obviously, it was necessary for me to work through my own feelings in respect to the terminal nature of a patient's illness. In any form of serious, individual psychotherapy, there is a constant communication between the unconscious of the patient and that of the therapist. If the therapist has unresolved feelings of futility or hopelessness due to the fact that he is working with a dying person, these feelings are likely to be communicated to the patient.

My approach in working with the terminally ill is

oriented toward life, and based on the belief that one can search for the fullest use of oneself under any conditions, no matter how painful and discouraging they are. I often give patients Victor Frankl's *From Death Camp to Existentialism* to read. In this book, Frankl describes his own inner growth and development during the time he was in the only hell ever devised by man that matches the hell of the cancer patient—the German concentration camps.

Because the cancer patient has usually lost the central relationship of his life even before the development of his cancer, he feels very much alone and isolated in a hostile and uncaring universe. The therapist, by his presence and by his real interest, can give the patient meaning through warm human contact, can, by providing the opportunity for a strong relationship, give the patient an anchor rope to the world and to others. With contact and connectedness returned, and with the focus on life rather than on death, the patient's fear of death seems to diminish considerably. Life takes on a reality and a sense of excitement as the search for the self proceeds. There is no longer an overwhelming sense of loss and isolation, but rather a feeling of commitment and involvement. The philosopher Kierkegaard wrote, "I need to discover the truth for me: something to hold on to although the world shatter about my ears." The truth for oneself is, indeed, a powerful aid in times of catastrophe. For the patient with a disastrous physical illness, its discovery is a tool that brings strength, composure and added physical ability to fight for life.

The reader will have gathered that the approach of crisis therapy is somewhat different from traditional psychotherapy. The methods I devised for working with terminal cancer patients are based on a number of concepts that need to be fully understood if the nature of crisis therapy is to be clear. There are five points on which psychoanalysis, and the therapies springing from it, have held a definite viewpoint that is different from that of crisis therapy. These five points are:

1. Psychic Determinism—Man As a Machine
2. The Basic Moral Nature of Man
3. The Nature of Mental Health
4. The Basic Question That Psychotherapy Should Try to Answer
5. The Best Way for One Human Being to Understand Another

In order to clarify the viewpoint of crisis therapy, I will first present the psychoanalytic assumption in their strongest (and perhaps most exaggerated) form, followed by my own assumption.

Since the seventeenth century there has been a gradual growth of the concept of the machine. The concept of "natural law" originally meant that certain observed events seemed invariably to follow each other—the freezing of water at a certain temperature, for instance. But this concept has gradually come to mean that all events could be viewed as determined, obeying rigidly sequential laws of cause and effect. The universe itself has become viewed as a giant machine.

Since psychology developed out of the same philo-sophical seed bed as the other sciences, it was only natural that the same basic orientation should be followed. Human behavior came to be viewed as though it were as completely determined as that of billiard balls; and it was believed that if we could understand the basic mathematical laws involved, we could predict and control human behavior as accurately as billiard balls. It was not only the cosmos that operated as a clockwork system, but also man himself. As pointed out in an earlier chapter, most cancer patients accept this view of the universe completely, but in an extremely negative way, in that they believe the hopelessness of their lives to be inevitable. That is one reason why traditional psychotherapy is ineffective with cancer patients. Part of their despair stems from the fact that they believe their lives to be fully determined. A therapeutic approach that shares this view cannot succeed in countering it.

It is true that human beings seemed more like elliptical billiard balls on a warped table—thus, it was recognized that human behavior was extremely complex. But the basic principle of man as a machine was implicitly accepted. This viewpoint permeated the field of psychology far more than is generally realized. For example, a recent study showed that psychological and psychiatric language has five times as many terms implying "passivity" and "being acted upon" as it has terms implying "action," "self-organization" and "self-steering behavior." The cancer patient, of course, sees himself as being acted upon; to regain his sense of

101

self, it is action and self-organization that is needed. Thus, once again, the difficulty of traditional approaches with the cancer patient become obvious.

The two extremes of psychology—psychoanalysis and conditioning theory—both held the man-as-machine assumption. Freud wrote, "We do not live; we are lived by unknown and uncontrollable forces." He pictured the helpless ego as harried this way and that between powerful drives from the unconscious and the rigid walls of the super-ego. Frec will was seen as an illusion. The other extreme of psychology—conditioning theory —held that if we could mathematically order the factors in the conditioning of human beings, we could absolutely predict and control human behavior.

Now, it is undeniably true that this approach to human behavior has yielded much knowledge and some results. For certain narrow areas of human behavior, it *has* advanced us and it *does* work. Certainly no understanding of human beings and no psychotherapy today would be valid without the knowledge brought to us by the exploitation of this concept. Yet we cannot explain in any satisfactory manner, by either a Freudian or a Pavlovian analysis of the data, such things as tragedy, beauty, courage, faithfulness, laughter, love or heroism. Nor can we help the terminally ill patient to fight for his life, if we approach the task from a mechanistic viewpoint. The "machine" that the human being inhabits, his body, has already been declared damaged beyond repair—as good as dead.

The humanistic psychologist Abraham Maslow put

it this way: "When one wishes knowledge of persons or societies, mechanistic science breaks down completely." On this fundamental issue, therefore, crisis therapy takes a completely different approach. Crisis therapy sees the human being as freest in the area where he is most healthy, where he is least bound by rigid needs from the past. The human individual is viewed as active, decision-making and free within limits—Paul Tillich uses the apt term "finite freedom"—and not as passive, controlled and determined. The patient is viewed as having at least as much free will and at least as much ability to transcend his unconscious defenses as does the therapist.

This approach stresses the dignity of the human being, his ability to learn, to master and transcend his unconscious drives, and to act on his decisions. Indeed, the strength and dignity of Freud's own life, his mastery of illness and pain, his refusal to make easy decisions, his searching beyond his own defenses for truth, and his immense courage, all contribute to my own view—as embodied in crisis psychotherapy—that there is more to the mind of man than unconscious forces that rigidly control a helpless ego.

The second assumption on which crisis psychotherapy differs from traditional approaches concerns the basic moral nature of human beings. The eighteenth and nineteenth centuries were marked by a great debate on this question. On one side was the Natural Man of

Thomas Hobbes, "nasty, brutish and cold." On the other was the Noble Savage of Jean Jacques Rousseau, "unspoiled by civilization." During the Victorian period, the combined effects of the Industrial Revolution and misunderstood Darwinism decided the argument in favor of Hobbes. Human beings came to be seen as essentially selfish, narcissistic, murderous, impulsive and, generally, not very nice. It was believed that it was up to civilization to restrain and control these elements of the Freudian id. Psychotherapy saw its task as the manipulation of personality so as to achieve the best, most painless and most efficient sublimations of the basic pathological drives.

In the past, among descriptions of patients and discussions of personality theory, it was difficult to find statements concerning positive psychological forces. In a psychiatric or psychological staff conference 25 years ago, when I began my work with cancer patients, the use of such terms as "courage," "strength" (unless speaking of ego-strength), "love," "compassion," or "determination" was to invite a hard time at the hands of one's colleagues. When I first became a therapist, I should make clear, my orientation was as traditional as you could find. But the more I worked with cancer patients, trying to deal with their special problems, the more I came to feel that the traditional approaches and views simply would not do. The negativistic aspects of traditional psychotherapy came to bother me more and more, and my own views changed greatly.

It came to disturb me greatly that, in the traditional

viewpoint, positive behavior should be seen as resulting merely from combinations of such ego-defense mechanisms as sublimation and over-compensation, and that positive drives were regarded as illusions, or reactions against negative drives. From that viewpoint, the painter is seen as basically seeking to sublimate his drives to smear feces—and so much for Rembrandt and Chagall. The search for God was the search for a lost father figure and thus philosophers such as Bruno and Spinoza were dismissed. The attempt to understand the universe and our place in it is seen as intellectualization or an attempt to find out what *really* went on in your parents' bedroom—and so much for Freud, Einstein and Aristotle.

This view has gone so far that there has been a loss of belief in the trustworthiness of the patient. Lawrence Brody refers to this reaction as the "Oho phenomenon": whenever the patient says something, the therapist responds with an inward, "Oho, I know what that means." Gordon Allport has described this as "a kind of contempt for the psychic surface of life. The individual's conscious report is rejected as untrustworthy and the contemporary thrust of his motives is disregarded in favor of a backward-tracing to earlier formative stages." Thus the patient loses his right to be believed.

Crisis psychotherapy rejects this viewpoint. I have based it, instead, on a belief that pathological drives emerge when the individual is frustrated in his attempt to achieve himself and to express his positive drives in his own unique way. Negative drives are seen as natural,

105

but as secondary rather than primary. Such negative drives as seen as becoming predominant in the individual only when his drive for self-actualization is frustrated. In Karen Horney's words, "We believe that man turns unconstructive or destructive only if he cannot fulfill himself."

The cancer patient, as we have seen, almost invariably is contemptuous of himself, and of his abilities and possibilities. He cannot be helped by suggesting that he sublimate his negative drives. Rather, his positive drives must be freed from the dark box in which they have been for so long shut away. He cannot be helped to view himself positively unless the therapist holds that view as well.

Carl Rogers has written, "One of the most revolutionary concepts to grow out of our clinical experiences is the growing recognition that the innermost core of man's nature, the deepest levels of his personality, the base of his "animal nature" is positive in character, is basically socialized, forward-moving, rational, and realistic." This fundamental statement, perhaps more than any other, sums up my viewpoint in developing crisis psychotherapy. The freer and more self-actualized the individual is, the more he will behave in ways that are socially as well as personally positive. The drive to complete and fulfill himself is seen as existing at the deepest levels of the individual. But for the individual's potential to be realized, there must be an outlet—and it is this outlet that the cancer patient has denied himself in his attempt to gain the love of others by being the person *they* wish him to be.

The third basic assumption on which the two approaches to therapy differ concerns the nature of "mental health." If one views man as a machine, it is fairly clear what health means: the machine must be kept in good "repair." A machine should be adjusted to its environment. It should not cause trouble or upset around it. It should conform to its environmental needs—in this case the cultural mores of the given society. And, since the analyst is a healer with a great tradition behind him, the machine should run with as little pain as possible. Thus, in traditional psychotherapy, mental health is considered to be a well-adjusted, symptom-free state in which the individual functions as efficiently as possible and with as little pain as possible.

This is not a goal to be lightly dismissed. All of us who have suffered from psychic pain know something of its value.

But the crisis psychotherapy definition of mental health is somewhat more complex. In crisis psychotherapy, therefore, I stress what Carl Rogers has called "an openness to experience—a willingness and desire to grow in our own natural, organic direction." No specific static position or goal is sought; the object of psychotherapy is seen as encouraging a zest for life, a zest for growing and developing. The approach is akin

107

to that of the gardener who wants his iris to become the best possible iris and the peony the best possible peony. For each individual in crisis psychotherapy, the goal is different. Each person is seen as having a special song to sing; a special rhythm to beat out in terms of his acting, reacting, relating and creating. When he sings his own song, he experiences a zest for life, an enjoyment of life, and a meaning in life.

The importance of this approach in working with cancer patients cannot be overstated. In most cases, the patient's despair arises out of the fact that he or she has not been singing his or her unique song. They have tried to sing other people's songs all their lives, and the effort has brought them only frustration and self-contempt. Nothing can be more important for them than to discover their own particular song and learn to project it loudly and clearly.

Sidney Jourard has written, "Healing is rooted in the structure of the total organism and the best the therapist can do is to cooperate with nature, that is, to help the organism function in its own way as effectively and completely as possible." From my own viewpoint, the crucial phrase in this statement is "in its own way." The goal is to help the patient become so fully at one with himself that he reacts spontaneously and fully in life. The patient's symptoms are viewed as the result of an inability to be himself freely, and also as behavior patterns which continue to block such open expression of the self. Maslow has put the issue quite bluntly: "It seems quite clear that personality problems may be loud protests against the crushing of one's psychological bones, of one's true nature."

In many of the case histories outlined in previous chapters, this crushing of the psychological bones stands out with the clarity of an x-ray photograph. The case of John, who wanted a musical career for himself, but became a lawyer to please his father, is particularly relevant here. For not only did John's despair leave him once he began to "sing his own song," but his supposedly terminal brain cancer went into remission. Gotthard Booth wrote, "Illness is a reminder of the purpose of life." And in John's case this was true to an astonishing extent. Told that he was going to die, John refused to give up; it was he himself who found out about and contacted the Institute of Applied Biology, where we were indeed able to help him fight successfully for his life. John's illness—and his recovery—related directly to his ability to express his true self. When he became totally blocked in the achievement of his basic goals of self-realization, deep depression engulfed him, followed by the development of cancer. But when he once again began to quest after the goals that alone could bring fulfillment to his natural self, both his psychological and his physical symptoms disappeared.

The reduction of symptoms as the individual learns who he is and tries to live honestly and fully in his own way applies both to the psychological and physical aspects of his being. The more he expresses his basic self in ways organic and natural to him, the healthier he tends to become on all levels. The less he is himself, the greater strain is placed on him, and the greater is the tendency to illness. In *Dr. Zhivago,* Boris Pasternak wrote:

> The great majority of us are required to live a life of constant, systematic duplicity. Your health is bound to be affected if, day after day, you say the opposite of what you feel, if you grovel before what you dislike and rejoice at what brings you nothing but misfortune. Our nervous system isn't just a fiction, it's a part of our physical body, and our soul exists in space and is inside us, like the teeth in our mouth. It cannot be forever violated with impunity.

If I am to help a patient to sing his own song, it is necessary to look for what is *right* with the patient. This need brings us directly to a fourth basic assumption in which crisis therapy differs from traditional approaches: the basic question psychotherapy should try to answer. In traditionally based therapies, the question is, "What is wrong with you?" As corollaries, two other questions are asked: "What caused this?" and "How can we get rid of the cause?" But for me, in crisis psychotherapy, the basic question is, "What is right with you?" And the corollary questions are: "What are your special ways of being, relating, acting, creating?" and "What is blocking their expression?"

The difference in these two basic questions causes a profoundly different atmosphere to prevail during therapy. To put it bluntly (and perhaps a bit unfairly, in order to make the point), how is a person going to feel about himself after a couple of years of searching for and concentrating on the things that are wrong with him? And how is he going to feel after a couple of years of searching for the things that are right with him?

Viewing man as a machine, the traditionally based therapies ask, "What is causing this specific machine to malfunction, and how can we find and repair or bypass the damaged part?" Viewing man as a striving, seeking and self-actualizing organism, crisis psychotherapy asks, "How can we help this individual to achieve himself in the fullest, richest way?" Although the two approaches use many of the same basic concepts—the great wealth of knowledge that Freud and his followers amassed— one school approaches the patient with the attitude of the mechanic, the other with the attitude of the gardener.

The final assumption on which the two approaches differ concerns the best way for people to get to know and understand one another. In traditional psycho- therapy, the great stress is on objectivity. The belief is that by observing with the cool detached eye of the scientist, the patient's difficulties can best be seen, and best be helped. Crisis psychotherapy does not accept this viewpoint. Instead, my belief is that while there must be some degree of objectivity, some ability to remain apart and see the total picture, real understanding of another person is gained only by interacting with that person, and responding to him as a complete self. From this viewpoint, it is necessary to love in order to understand.

Sidney Jourard, in his book *The Transparent Self*, describes one aspect of this need for meeting the patient fully: "Surely our patients come to us because they have become so estranged from their real selves, that they are incapable of making these known to their associates in life. I do not see how we can reacquaint our patients with their real selves by striving to subject them to subtle manipulations and thus to withhold our real selves from them. It reminds me of the sick leading the sick."

To react spontaneously and wholeheartedly with the patient is not the same thing, however, as reacting in a naïve manner. We might use the example of two automobile drivers in traffic. Both act spontaneously, but one has been driving a week, and the other for five years. The difference is obvious. In crisis psychotherapy, then, the therapist's spontaneity is real. It is also a spontaneity that is experienced, trained, committed and knowledgeable. Because the therapist is entering as a person into the therapeutic encounter, ethics and values enter with him. In the traditionally based therapies, a real attempt was made to keep ethics and values out of the therapy. In crisis psychotherapy, a real attempt is made to include them.

Clark Moustakas—whose approach is very close to my own—has spoken of progress in psychotherapy as occurring "not through arrangement of conditions, not through pre-determined goals, or criteria for evaluation, but through genuine encounters which in their very nature are spontaneous, unpredictable, and unique."

From this viewpoint, therapy sessions are not planned—they occur. They are unpredictable, vital, alive. By meeting the patient fully as a person, I try to tempt the patient to meet me; by doing so, the patient may eventually come to meet *himself* as well.

The question is not, "What should I do to this patient to heal him?" Rather, in Carl Roger's phrase, it is, "How can I provide a relationship which this person may use for his own personal growth?" As a crisis psychotherapist, I am not at the ready to "interpret" every statement the patient makes. I believe it is necessary to listen, and to accept the possibility the patient knows what he is talking about. I accept the likelihood that the shoe is pinching as much in the present as it did in the patient's childhood, and that the patient may be speaking realistically, not symbolically. The typical cancer patient has, after all, always feared to reveal his true self, convinced that that self is unacceptable. If the patient is allowed to feel that the therapist does not believe his statements to be the full truth, but that they "mean something else," then the patient's feeling of hopelessness will only be reinforced. Thus the objectivity that is the hallmark of traditional therapies can only stand in the way of helping the cancer patient. An open encounter in both directions is essential to the restoration of the patient's self-esteem.

In this chapter I have presented five basic philosophical assumptions on which crisis therapy differs

113

strongly from psychoanalysis. Obviously, these differences lead to many alternative psychotherapeutic techniques. These techniques will be presented in detail in the next two chapters. In addition, a number of these techniques will serve as the basis for methods that the reader can make use of to combat the kinds of emotional constriction that create fertile ground for the development of cancer.

It should be pointed out here that the techniques of crisis therapy were used not only with my patients who had cancer, but also with the cancer-free control group. The control group consisted of 88 patients whom I saw individually for a total of more than 8,000 hours of psychotherapy. They comprised the usual type of patients seen in office practice in a large city. These patients also responded very positively to crisis therapy. They seemed to move much faster and more easily than patients whom I had previously treated with techniques based upon traditional psychoanalytic philosophical assumptions. Thus the questions that I had to ask myself in trying to help cancer patients learn to fight for their lives, led me to understand in new ways the nature of the psychotherapeutic encounter as a whole.

I Want to Live 7

During my seventh therapy session with Donald, the following dialogue took place:

> *Donald:* I'm afraid of my cancer. I want to live.
>
> *LeShan:* Why? Whose life do you want to live?
>
> *Donald:* I detest it! I've never lived my own life. There was always so much to do at the moment. So much to . . . I never got around to living my life.
>
> *LeShan:* You never even were able to find out what it was.

Donald: That's why I drink. It makes things look better. Not so dark.

LeShan: Maybe the better way would be to find out what is your way of life and start living it.

Donald: How could I do that?

LeShan: That's what we're trying to do here.

As discussed in the previous chapter, "your way of life" is different for each patient. But the goal is always the same: to mobilize the resources of the total being in ways that will rekindle the creative life forces. In spite of a great deal of work in the fields of philosophy, psychology and psychiatry, a useful way of conceptualizing the life and death forces in the individual has not as yet been formulated. From both clinical and experimental data we know that the "desire to live" is variable between different individuals and, to a lesser extent, within the same individual at different periods in his life. We know also that this variation can have profound effects on the resistance of the total organism to stress and to disease processes. Psychological factors related to the desire to live can under certain conditions provide the individual with an almost unbelievable ability to cope with illness or stress—or, on the other hand, can so weaken the individual that he dies despite the lack of observable physical reasons.

For terminal cancer patients, as we have seen, life has been dominated by a problem they must solve but cannot. The failure of the life force is usually connected to this unsolved problem. One patient, in speaking of a period five years before the first signs of her cancer said, "If I looked ahead in life, there was nothing I could see unless I kidded myself." Another patient, at the beginning of therapy, put it this way: "What I really wanted in life is impossible for me ever to have. What I can have I don't really want. There never really was a way out for me." A third patient had a favorite saying that, it seemed to her, symbolized her whole life: "If the rock drops on the egg—poor egg. If the egg drops on the rock—poor egg." It is this fundamental attitude that the therapist must come to grips with—and as quickly as possible.

A patient may wish to live and fight for life for different reasons. Donald, the patient quoted at the beginning of this chapter, expressed the two most frequent reasons in the same breath: the fear of death ("I'm afraid of my cancer"), and the desire to live ("I want to live"). But clinical experience indicates rather strongly that in cases of serious physical illness, the fear of death is not a very powerful tool. The fear of death does not appear to bind the resources of the individual together, or to increase resistance to the disease processes. Certainly, it does not help the patient expand his personality to fulfill his potential. On the contrary, it restricts and binds him. The fear of death is an essentially negative emotion. The wish to live is a much stronger weapon, positive and liberating. It gives patient and therapist something to work toward together.

But how can the wish to live be fully revived in those

117

who feel defeated by life? Like Donald, even as they say, "I want to live," they revile the actual life they have lived and are living. Therefore, in mobilizing the wish to live we must first have goals in the future which are deeply important to the patient. We need an ideal to work toward. Maslow has pointed out that each culture has its ideal individual. These include the "hero," "saint," "mystic," "gentleman," and others. In our time, we tend to have given up these ideals, however. We strive to be "well-adjusted." But the ideal of being well-adjusted has little pull-value toward the future. Who would work hard and long, suffer pain, fight for life, in order to be merely "well-adjusted"?

The ideal of the full rich self, however, of developing one's own being in one's own special way, of achieving the freedom to be fully oneself without fear—that is a goal that is acceptable within our culture and also worth fighting and suffering for. It is a goal literally worth living for. The problem, of course, is that most cancer patients have long since given up hope for attainment of the self. Generally, they have judged and condemned their inner self, believing it to be unacceptable.

The following interchange took place with Joan, early in her therapy:

> *LeShan:* Isn't it time you started being concerned about you, and stopped being concerned about people's reactions to you?
>
> *Joan:* But they're important. That's our job. What I have to do.

> *LeShan:* Sometimes one's job is to cultivate one's garden. The garden in one's backyard, in the front, or the one in one's heart.
>
> *Joan:* What's the use of cultivating a little patch of rocks surrounded by high, thick hedges?
>
> *LeShan:* That's how you see your heart?
>
> *Joan:* Yes.

To a patient who feels this way about herself, it is not enough to say, "You have every reason to live," even when the assertion is buttressed by a list of the patient's perceived assets. The deep concern and involvement with life which is central to the wish to live cannot be aroused by logic and reason. The approach must go deeper—bringing an arousal of faith in the self and concern with the self. The patient's despair must be countered by something as deep as itself. The therapist's faith in the patient must be strong enough to overcome the patient's acceptance of despair.

When I write here of "faith" in the patient, the term is used in the sense of Paul Tillich's statement, "Faith is the state of being ultimately concerned." Ultimate concern means primary concern. Other concerns—the therapist's concern for himself and his own ego, for his hurt if the patient dies, for his own pride—must be secondary, and sometimes sacrificed. The therapist's faith must of course be real—it cannot be faked.

This is one of the reasons that the patient load—the number of terminally ill patients—must be kept small. When I began my work with cancer patients, there was a period when *all* my patients were terminally ill and I was working fourteen hours a day. This situation proved to be an enormous strain. The nature of crisis therapy required that I give myself as fully and openly as possible to each patient. But none of us can give and give without surcease. To try to do so, I found, was bad for me and bad for my patients. I remember, vividly and with pain, sitting in Joan's hospital room and being unable to truly help her. She was close to death. I knew it and she knew it. But because of the strain of having so many cancer patients, and of the deaths of so many people I loved, I had become, temporarily, a "burnt-out case," to use Graham Greene's phrase. At that point Joan needed warm human contact more than she ever had, but I had allowed myself to become so drained that in spite of every effort I would make, I could be there in that room only as a hollow shell and not as a human being. Joan realized that, and it confirmed her worst suspicions about herself and her life. That was unquestionably the worst moment in all my work with cancer patients. I was failing Joan just as she had always expected to be failed.

That experience taught me, once and for all, that I could not help more than a few terminally ill patients at once. I do not believe that any therapist can. It is essential for those undertaking therapy with cancer victims to have other kinds of patients as well. Even so, the emotional drain is considerable. Thus it is vital that the therapist be aware of his own inner resources and their limits. Once one starts to work with a patient who is terminally ill, it is not easy to stop in the middle;

if therapy is abandoned, it is likely to precipitate a strong depressive reaction. It is better, in fact, not to start at all than to start and not finish. "Who rides the tiger, cannot dismount," goes the old saying. Equally, who enters a commitment with a dying patient, cannot abandon it. (During the first year of therapy with a particular cancer patient, the therapist's vacations—and I can attest that they are absolutely necessary—must be carefully prepared for. Where other types of patients may feel anxiety, cancer patients often show negative biological changes. The therapist must be prepared and prepare for this.)

The goal of crisis therapy is well expressed in the story of the Chassidic mystic Rabbi Zusia, who said: "When I die, God will not ask me why I was not Moses. He will ask me why I was not Zusia." Most cancer patients, as we have seen, have rejected their true selves; and at the same time they have set impossible demands upon themselves, so that they might not even be satisfied to be Moses himself. Like Virginia, whose words were quoted in Chapter Four, even to win the Miss Universe title and have all future contests called off would not be enough to convince such patients of their worthiness.

Yet the very fact that a patient is suffering from a *terminal* illness opens the way to helping them. There is, for one thing, a greater willingness on the part of the patient to accept the possibilities of psychotherapy. Having been told that death is imminent, there is less reason for these patients to fight against the revelation of their true selves—it sometimes appears that they do not fear to reveal the true self as much because they do not expect to live long enough to have to cope with the consequences of doing so. One patient, for instance, had been told that he had a fatal malignancy and was going to die by a certain date. Under a new type of chemotherapy treatment, his cancer diminished and disappeared. As he was about to be discharged from the hospital, he said to his physician: "Doctor, you may not be aware of it, but my biggest problem was not that I was going to die. It's what to do with my life now that I've recovered." Such patients have so lost contact with their own inner resources, the original springs from which their desires flow, that they seem to say, in Samuel Beckett's words:

Where would I go, if I could go, who would I be,
if I could be, what would I say if I had a voice,
who says this, saying it's me?

But now that the battle against themselves appears to be over, they are willing to drop their guard slightly. A chink is opened in their armor. In addition, there appears to be a freshening need to "set their house in order," a certain fatalistic curiosity as to *why* they have never managed to come to terms with themselves. This curiosity is not always openly expressed, but it is there, and it gives the therapist one more possibility on which to build. Curiosity is not yet understanding or acceptance —but it is fertile ground in which to plant the seeds of full celebration of the self.

Thus, I found that if I could communicate to the patient my own faith in human possibility, and my dedication to finding that well-spring in the patient himself, the patient usually is willing to go along. I can achieve this communication, however, only by meeting, *encountering* the patient in such a full, honest manner that the patient *knows* who I am and what I honestly believe. If a patient asks me my opinion or feeling about a subject, I say what I truly think. In this work there can be no hiding place, no mask for concealment on the part of either the therapist or the patient. The issues are too great, the stakes too high, for halfway measures. I found that I must break through the wall that generally separates people and become fully "engaged" with the patient. Carl Rogers explains it this way:

> I have found that the more I can be genuine in a relationship, the more helpful it is. This means that I need to be aware of my own feelings, in so far as possible, rather than presenting an outward façade of one attitude, while actually holding another attitude at a deeper or unconscious level. Being genuine also involves the willingness to be and to express, in my words and behavior, the various feelings and attitudes which exist in me. It is only in this way that the relationship can have *reality,* and the reality seems deeply important as a first condition. It is only by providing the genuine reality which is in me that the other person can successfully seek the reality in him.

123

You Can Fight for Your Life

Honesty on the part of the therapist is of crucial importance. A lie between patient and therapist (even if the patient does not "catch" the therapist at it) quickly destroys any validity the therapy has, and turns it into a mere discussion of permissible subjects between acquaintances. With one exception, all my patients knew that their condition was considered medically hopeless. The exception was Judith, a lovely, bright 24-year-old woman. Her family had approached me and said that Judith wanted psychotherapy, that they had heard of my work and would like to have her see me, but only on the condition that I would agree not to tell her that she had cancer.

I accepted, but with great misgivings. Judith told me that she was there to discuss personal and marital problems. She added that she had an arthritic back condition that occasionally gave her pain, but that radiation seemed to help. In spite of mutual liking and respect between us, little progress was made for several months. Insight and understanding did not seem to produce any change in feeling or behavior on Judith's part. Then she began to have dreams, as well as waking feelings, of being followed by something dangerous. Her sense of anxiety and isolation gradually increased. More and more of her psychic energy seemed to be needed to hold the knowledge of her condition at unconscious levels. Clearly she knew that something was seriously wrong, but did not want to admit it to herself.

With much trepidation, I called her husband and told him that I was going to tell Judith the truth on my next visit. I said that my responsibility was to her and not to any promises I had been stupid enough to make to the family. He agreed to be waiting outside the office in his car after the appointment. When I started to discuss her "back condition" at our next session, Judith was resistant and uncomfortable. Obviously, she wanted to change the subject. I persisted, described the condition, named it, and told her that while it was very serious, much could and would be done to try to control it—no one was "giving her up" or abandoning hope. She listened carefully and asked thoughtful, intelligent questions. She did not seem depressed as she left.

At the next session she told me, "When you started to talk about my illness last week, I was very angry with you. I still felt resentful in the car on the way home. Then suddenly it seemed as if a tremendous weight had been lifted from my shoulders. I felt better and more relaxed than I have in months."

She went on to say that during the intervening week, she and her husband had become closer and talked more than they had in many months. The sense of isolation and anxiety vanished and did not reappear for the year and a half that she lived beyond that time. Therapy began to make real progress and she was able to do and enjoy things that had never been possible for her previously.

The mistake of lying to a patient—or joining in a conspiracy to lie—I made only this once. All my other patients either knew the true picture before treatment or were relieved to hear the truth—and discuss it openly—when told of their condition at the first session. No other approach, I believe, is worth undertaking, for if the therapist does not tell the truth, he will only succeed in communicating to the patient his own fear of what the patient fears, and his inability to cope with the true situation.

Honesty cannot be limited, of course, to such fundamental questions; it must permeate the relationship between therapist and patient at all levels. The honesty of the encounter precludes kindness. Kindness in most cases involves not only a self-protective shield for the therapist himself, but also implies a superior position. Empathy, not sympathy, is needed. And the empathy must go both ways. One must be in full contact with the patient before the patient can accept being in contact with his or her own self and life.

An analogy can be made with a psychotherapeutic problem that arises in working very intensively with schizophrenics. Between the unconscious of the therapist and the unconscious of such patients there is only the therapist's ego. The therapist is in danger of being drawn into a schizophrenic reality. In crisis therapy, there is a deliberate attempt to reverse this process. Here there is only one defensive system between the patient's ego and the therapist's ego—the defensive system of the patient. The patient is thus in "danger" of being drawn into the world he basically wants to enter so very much, yet is afraid to.

The naked encounter between patient and therapist makes it clear to the cancer patient that the therapist accepts him without reservation, and therefore without fear. The patients can thus begin to question their own fears of encountering themselves. It is not until this "meeting" is accomplished that the process of psychotherapy becomes real to the cancer patient. Without such a meeting, patients may often be cooperative and work hard, but the patient remains untouched at his or her vital center.

It is indicative of the openness of the encounter that patients have frequently felt free to point out my own errors of judgment. I have, in fact, learned much from them. One patient, for instance, said, "You have a habit that always annoys me. At the end of each session you summarize what we've done and learned. If I haven't got an idea already, I'm not going to get it when you beat it to death at the end. Probably this is right for some patients, but not for me." She was right. I realized that I did have this habit, having generalized it from several patients with whom it had proved useful.

As I pointed out in the previous chapter, this type of open encounter is directly contrary to much of the orientation of psychotherapy in the past. We had been trained *not* to meet the patient openly and fully, but rather to hide behind our professional masks, observing and reacting *to* the patient instead of interacting *with* him. But without such interaction the patient will never be convinced that the therapist does truly care, does have faith. And unless the patient is convinced of this, he will not be willing to begin the encounter with himself that alone can mobilize his will to live.

I should make it plain, in this context, that I have never had a patient ask me an untactful personal question or one that I would have preferred not to answer.

An acceptance of my right to privacy has been universal. But the patient's privacy is also respected. It is made clear very early in therapy that the patient does *not* have to tell the therapist everything, that he has a right to privacy and that if he does not want to discuss a particular subject, he can say so and shift the discussion.

This "right to privacy" may seem to contradict the idea of the open encounter. In fact, it buttresses it. By giving the patient the right to privacy, the patient's sense of himself as an adult, rather than as the therapist's symbolic child, is enhanced. An attitude of respect for the patient as an adult has the additional purpose of preventing the formation of a transference neurosis. Since the therapist is "transparent" and therefore perceived realistically as a person with short-comings as well as strengths, he does not serve as a shadow-screen on which the patient can project his unconscious needs. A realistic dependency—as on a guide who "knows the route"—is formed instead. One measurement of progress in therapy, a measurement of which both participants should be aware, is the gradual loss of this dependency and a corresponding new growth toward full selfhood on the part of the patient.

Judith summed up this relationship well when she sent me a Christmas card on which she had written: "Thank you for being my ally." She did not mean an ally in her conflicts with others, but in the battle for her own full being. Another patient said very cheerfully one day, "You know, Joe [her fiancé] is now much more useful than you are to discuss work problems with, and

May [a long-time friend with whom a much closer relationship had been formed recently than had previously existed] is better for talking about Joe. It looks like I'm beginning to phase you out." We both agreed that these were real steps on the road to our goals in therapy. This patient was not only saying, "I want to live," but was clearly beginning to find the ways in which she could live most fully.

I have said that the honesty required for crisis therapy precludes kindness. It also precludes carefulness. The approach cannot be cautious or tentative. Moustakas has pointed out the careful person is only one step away from the paltry person. Crisis therapy needs intense concentration, almost absolute caring and acceptance, but not carefulness. If the therapist has reservations about meeting the patient fully, the patient quickly senses them, reinforcing his reservations about meeting himself. But if the encounter can be made without carefulness on the therapist's side, and without second thoughts, the breakdown of the wall between the patient and his own inner resources will begin.

Psychotherapy, for the patient who is involved in a life and death struggle, cannot deal only with the technical aspects of the personality as they are found in the textbooks. The larger questions are too pressing, too imminent. Values MUST be explored. As Alma put it, "Once the big questions are asked, you can't forget them. You can only ignore them as long as no one raises them." Death, the figure in the background, asks the questions, and the therapist must join in the search for

129

answers that are meaningful to the patient. In the next chapter, I will be illustrating in detail the methods used in that search. A number of these techniques can also be used to help those persons whose personality patterns and life history might make them especially vulnerable to cancer, even though the disease has not yet struck.

These techniques, in general, are designed to help the patient discover his true values—in terms of who he is, what kind of person he is, and what type of relationships would make the most sense and be the most rewarding and satisfying to him. For when a patient has denied his true values, and has sought to be loved only on other people's terms, then life inevitably comes to seem a series of endless frustrations and disappointments—disappointment not only with others but also with the self. And the will to live, smothered by self-contempt, can all too easily become enveloped in despair.

If the will to live is to flourish, the individual must live according to his own values, and seek to be loved for his own self. This value system is beautifully expressed in the following poem put into the mouth of St. Francis by the Greek novelist Kazantzakis:

> I said to the almond tree
> "Sister, speak to me of God,"
> And the almond tree blossomed.

The Third Road 8

After several sessions with Betty, a woman in her early twenties who had Hodgkin's disease, I offered her the following interpretation of the things she had said about herself over the previous weeks:

"You feel as if there are only two possible roads for you in life and you have to choose one of them. The first road is being yourself and expressing yourself as you feel at the moment. It's being spontaneous and emotional and warm and loving, and letting others see who you are and how you feel. But you are sure that if you do this, everyone will withdraw from you and reject you,

131

and you will be all alone. The second road is to be a 'good girl,' like mother wants you to be, and to mind your manners and always do exactly what is expected of you, and conform to the wishes of the world and Mrs. Grundy. Never to express yourself freely, but always to be conscious of others' wishes and expectations. If you follow this second road, people will accept you and love you and take care of you. But since nobody will know how you feel or who you are, they won't be loving you but a mask, and so you will be just as much alone, really, as if you had taken the first road."

At this point, I saw that Betty was sitting on the edge of her seat, leaning forward and listening with great intensity, focusing on every word. She was clearly tremendously *involved* with what was being said. I continued:

"However, these two are not the only alternatives for you. There is a third road."

In a harsh, anguished tone, as though the words were being torn out of her, this usually calm and placid young woman cried out, "What is it?"

Another patient, Ben, who was 48, was given a similar interpretation of his basic attitude in our sixth session:

"So you feel that every time you act and talk in a way that reveals who you *really* are and how you *really* feel, you get criticized and treated with anger and contempt. And this makes you feel very strongly what you have always felt about yourself—that you are no good, a terrible person, and that you'd be better off dead. But if you talk or act in ways others seem to want you to, they respect and admire you and you feel depressed and hopeless and wish you were dead. And these are the only two ways you know to act or talk, and you feel there is no way out."

Ben replied, "That's it exactly. No matter what I do, I know I can't win. All my life I've tried and tried and it never works and never can work, and I've always known that the slogan was, Christ you can't win. No matter what I do. I'm not superstitious or stupid or saying, 'Somebody up there hates me.' That's just the way it is with me."

All of us, at one time or another, may be faced with a temporary situation in which we feel that no third road exists. It does, of course, but we may be unable to see it. The cancer-prone personality, however, *always* has that feeling: it is a fundamental aspect of his total approach to life. And that is why he is in despair.

In dealing with despair, I believe it is vital to make it clear at the start that I comprehend the patient's world-view, and that I understand how it came to be. But I must make it equally clear that this world-view is false —that the problem can be solved. Furthermore, I emphasize that the solution lies in the patient, and not in the outside situation. If the patient can find, accept, and give expression to the rejected part of himself, then others will accept him and respond to him positively. But to do this, the patient must first understand that he *has* in fact rejected himself.

You Can Fight for Your Life

It is often a problem to help the patient realize just how thoroughly he has rejected himself, and how much he is out of contact with his real feelings. One patient, Arlene, told me that I didn't know what I was talking about when I said that she had not only accepted her parents' rejection of her, but also agreed with it. I asked her to recall the incident in childhood in which she felt she had been most unfairly treated and hurt. She recalled an incident, and was able to visualize it in great detail. At the end of the incident she had been crying alone in her room. Arlene was able to "see" this scene quite clearly, and even described the clothes she had been wearing. I asked her to imagine that we had a "time machine" in the office. She was to get into it and, in her present adult person, travel back to that room and moment in her childhood.

> *LeShan:* You now enter—as you are now—the room in which little Arlene is crying on the bed. You walk into the room. She looks up at you. What do you do?
> *Arlene:* I'd hit her!

The amazement and shock that Arlene experienced on hearing herself say this was the first step toward a major re-orientation to her rejected self.

This "time machine" technique was essentially borrowed from Arthur Laurents' superb play, *A Clearing in the Woods*. It has proven quite useful in crisis therapy.

Through its use, patients will frequently begin to really understand that they have lost part of themselves, that they are not whole, and that *they can heal their own wounds* by accepting the child within themselves.

A rough measure of progress can be made by using this technique at intervals, with the same or with different childhood incidents. Both the patient and myself observe the reaction to the rejected self. This procedure was used several times with John. Each time he "explained" to the child he had been that everything would be all right, and that there was nothing to fear. It was a cool, teacher-student type of relationship that he established with this rejected self each time he was asked to visualize the situation. Then one day he brought in a dream.

"There was a long dock going out into the water," he said. "There were people on the shore, but no one on the dock except for a small boy on the very end. He was frightened of falling in and was crying. I was walking out on the dock toward him. I don't know why I was walking there. When I came near him, he started to run toward me. I knelt down and held out my arms. He ran into them and I stood up. As I carried him back toward the shore he stopped crying. I felt I loved him." As John finished relating this dream, we looked across at one another. The tears were flowing down both our faces. For John, as for so many other patients, a great change took place when he finally began to love the rejected child that he had been. That child was no longer "out there." An empty space that had always existed in him was finally filled—an empty space exactly the size of the child that had been.

It was shortly after this that John once more took up the music he had abandoned twice in his life in order to please his parents and his wife. As has been noted before, John now plays with a symphony orchestra, and the inoperable brain tumor that brought him to the institute to begin with has been in remission for many years. Having realized that he in fact loved the child who wanted to be a musician and not a lawyer like his father, and having recognized that everything was not going to be all right unless that rejected child was accepted as his true self, John mobilized the will to live to a truly powerful extent, and fought successfully for his life against all medical odds.

Stuart, another patient, eventually came to accept the self he had rejected in terms similar to John. When the "time machine" technique was used, Stuart recalled lying in bed as a child listening to his father's footsteps in the hall. His father, going past Stuart's room, went in to his older brother's room to chat with him for awhile before he went to sleep. This older brother, whose interests and personality were much closer to the father's than Stuart's, was much preferred by their father. Stuart remembered lying alone, feeling terribly sad. Because of his father's rejection, Stuart said he had felt that "I must have done something terrible." But he could not imagine what it was: "I guess I felt that it was just being *me* that was so terrible."

I asked Stuart what he would feel like doing, opening the door and looking in on himself, as the child he had been gazed up expectantly from the bed. He replied: "Going out and closing the door behind me, I guess. There's nothing to say to him at all."

Some forty hours of therapy later, the same scene was visualized once again. Asked the same question—what he would feel like doing on opening the door—Stuart looked at me indignantly and said: "Take him in my arms and hug him, of course. What else would you do with a poor kid like that?"

With Maureen, an extremely intelligent and able woman who had been a journalist, the technique was carried a step further, at Maureen's own suggestion. She chose a scene when she had been 10 years old, but found that the child she tried to "meet" was as suspicious of her as she was of the "child." To break down this barrier between her present and her past, Maureen conceived the idea of getting to know the child she had been by interviewing her in depth and then writing the interviews up. As this process of getting in touch with herself continued, Maureen found herself becoming more and more at ease with the child self she had rejected, and therefore more and more in contact with her present inner life, so much of which she had hidden from herself.

Indirect as well as direct methods can be used to help the patient get back in touch with his or her true desires and to re-establish the hope that has been thrown

137

away along with those desires. I found, for instance, that it was often useful to have patients read the Arthur Laurents play from which I had borrowed the "time machine" concept. It presents in clear and beautiful form the process of the search for the self. As I have mentioned before, Hermann Hesse's great novel *Steppenwolf* can also be helpful to cancer patients. After reading it, Judith said, "I didn't understand what it was all about, but after I finished it, I couldn't stop crying for two hours." Clearly, even though she had not entirely grasped it on an "intellectual" level, its emotional significance had come through strongly. Later, in referring to the meeting between the two parts of the novel's hero —Henry Haller and the wolf of the title—she told me she had been struck by the fact "that the wolf had such beautiful eyes and was sad. I guess maybe what I've hated so in me also has beautiful eyes and is sad."

The mere recognition of the fact that a part of the self has indeed been rejected is a major step forward for these patients. Often it is the first step toward understanding that a third road does exist. Sometimes the patient himself will discover a work of art or life situation that suddenly opens a door to understanding. One patient called my attention to Fellini's film *Juliet of the Spirits*. "Larry, you better see this film," he said. "It's exactly what you have been talking about. Somebody is stealing your stuff!"

The film does indeed parallel many of the concerns of crisis therapy. Fellini shows Juliet leading a barren life until she is thrown into an existential crisis by the infidelity of her husband. She meets and learns about the parts of herself that she has never accepted. These aspects of herself take the form of fantasy projections of a variety of strange but beguiling characters. Finally, she accepts and embraces these repressed elements of her personality. As the projections vanish, they murmur a last sentence to her: "Now you will never be alone." She is complete and strong at last. The fact that the outside environment has not changed is not important. *She* has changed. She has *become* herself.

I have talked to psychologists, psychiatrists and social workers who did not understand this movie, but I have never found a cancer patient who did not completely comprehend it. The person suffering from a catastrophic illness sometimes seems more open to the meanings of artistic creations—at least those that deal with despair and the loss of self—than do the healthy professionals who seek to help the patient.

Once the patient realizes how much he has condemned and rejected his inner self, it is sometimes useful to discuss this process in terms of a metaphorical trial. In his childhood, the patient in effect held a trial in which he was judge, jury and defendant. At this trial, on the basis of half-understood evidence and a child's limited understanding, he condemned himself as guilty. Having long forgotten that this trial ever took place, the patient has been responding to himself on the basis of that false verdict. The psychotherapy is a re-trial, this time with a defense attorney—two adults taking a fresh look at the evidence, trying to find out what kind of crime could have been committed by a child to merit such a severe rejection.

As part of this re-trial it is vital to ask the patient, and ask repeatedly, what he or she really wants in life. The central question of crisis therapy is: "What do *you* want to do with your life?" It is a question that must be asked in as many ways as the therapist can devise until the patient becomes oriented to its validity. Eleanor, for instance, at first spoke only of her illness—breast cancer —and her wish not to die. I asked her, "If you were completely well physically, would you want to go on living with your husband or would you prefer living alone?" Eleanor started to answer, stopped, looked puzzled and said with much surprise in her voice, "I don't know." From this point on she was able to work much more seriously on her psychotherapy and appeared to be in much better spirits.

The crucial nature of the question, "What do you want?" is illustrated by the example of another woman, Vivian, who terminated therapy rather than deal with the consequences of accepting herself and her own desires. When she told me that she wished to stop seeing me, I said that she had every right to make that choice and would respect it, but that if she could help me to understand why, I might be able to be more effective in trying to help other patients. Vivian replied, "No, it's not you, it's me. I understand what you are doing, and if I go on with you, I'll have to look at my marriage. If I look at it, I'll lose it, and if it's a choice between my marriage and my life, I'd rather lose my life."

This was the only patient who did leave therapy. I regretted her decision deeply, but the honesty essential to crisis therapy prevented me from saying to her, "We don't know that," or some other soothing remark. For she was right; she had grasped the situation exactly. But although she made a choice that went against herself, it was an aware choice. She had once again found herself "guilty," but she had rendered this new verdict as an adult who understood its consequences, not as a bewildered child.

The remainder of my patients, however, were willing to go on searching for the sometimes difficult answers to the hard questions involved in crisis psychotherapy. No matter how hard the questions, the patient must be pushed. Kindness must be put aside. If the patient is to have any possibility of overcoming the cancer that has invaded the body, the fight must begin at once. If the patient is to achieve any sense of the self, and thus derive any true pleasure, any renewed hope, during the time that is left, the fight must begin at once. The hard .questions must be asked, over and over again.

What do *you* want?

Often, what the patient truly wants is to fulfill just that part of himself or herself that has been rejected, whose wishes and impulses are regarded as unacceptable. Joan, who had a deep love of nature, and a great understanding of flowers and gardens, had rejected this aspect of herself because she believed only "intellectual" pursuits to be valid. She felt that her love of gardening was something shameful and childish. Because she did not read the latest professional journals and was not interested in discussing abstract theories, she felt inferior. Having tried to make herself in an image that she believed others would admire, she had lost touch with the most genuine and talented aspects of herself. Another patient had been a successful actress, and felt completely at home and at ease only on the stage. She had given it up, however—acting, she said was ". . . like children dressing up in their parents' clothes and pretending." Since her professional retirement, her life had consisted of a constant social whirl, arguments with her husband and an empty feeling of uselessness and hopelessness.

In helping patients to combat their feelings of shame, shame that had led them to reject the most creative aspects of themselves, another film proved to be useful. This is the French movie *The Shameless Old Lady*. With exquisite sensitivity, the actress Sylvie portrays an old woman who all her life had done the things she was supposed to do. She married, cared for her husband, raised her children, ran the house. Then after her husband's death, she begins to find out what *she* enjoys doing. She eats when she is hungry, goes for a walk in the middle of the night to watch the harbor lights, joins a group of local radicals, wanders in department stores, befriends a young woman of disrepute, buys a small car, goes on picnics with her new friends—of whom her grown children strongly disapprove—and generally enjoys life and lives it more fully during her last 18 months than she has ever done before. As a picture of the kind of attitude toward life that crisis therapy tries to bring about, and as an answer to the question, "What's the use at my age?" *The Shameless Old Lady* is wonderfully evocative. It is her family—other people—who think her shameless. To herself, she is a heroine. And so, indeed, is she to the viewer.

Yet even when the cancer patient comes to the point of accepting the "shameful" rejected self, and begins to say, "Yes, this is what *I* want to do," there is the further difficulty of actually beginning to do it. It often seems to patients that their goals are so large, so overwhelmingly difficult to attain, that it is hopeless even to make the attempt. A technique taught me by Ensor Holiday for handling this problem has been very useful. This is the "first thing" technique. Once a goal is defined, the therapist keeps asking, "To accomplish that, what is the *first thing* you have to do?" General answers are not accepted and the question is repeated until the answer is a specific, single, concrete act that can be *done*. One of Holiday's patients, for instance, wanted to travel to France, but regarded the trip as impossible. Finally, after 11 repetitions of the question, the patient said, "First, I have to buy a new pair of shoelaces." This may seem insignificant to the point of amusement, but in fact it *was* the first step in his going to France.

One of the values of this re-orientation technique is that it helps train patients to think in terms of *action* to achieve their inner goals. Thinking in terms of action in itself makes the goal seem more real, possible and justified. If one can act in terms of a goal—no matter

143

how small the action may be—one has already begun
to accept as valid the idea that the goal can be achieved.
The action (or even concretizing the action verbally)
trains a person to begin to think that it is legitimate to
have such goals.

One of my patients, Abigail, had hated her profession
for 20 years, even though she was very successful at it.
Yet she had always felt it was impossible to change her
career. In therapy, she found out what she really wanted
to do, but to her it was merely an impossible dream.
After nearly 20 repetitions of the question, "What is the
first thing to do?" she finally decided that it was to buy
a stamp on her way home—in order to send for a college catalogue to find out if certain evening courses were
available. Abigail eventually went on to change careers.
Her new job paid half as much as her former position,
and carried with it far less social prestige. But she had
found herself; she was giving creative expression to the
rejected self that she had despised all her adult life. In her
new career she was happy and fulfilled. Five years after
her terminal malignancy was first diagnosed, she wrote
to me that she was too busy to worry about cancer: "I
simply do not have time," she said, "for that sort of
nonsense."

The Chinese have a saying: "The longest journey is
started by putting out your left foot." By repeatedly asking which foot is the left one—"What do *you* really
want?"—the therapist makes plain his belief in the
validity of the journey and the ability of the patient to
complete it. Abigail is proof that the journey can in-

deed be made. It is now ten years since her malignant melanoma, already widely spread, was first diagnosed, and she is indeed too busy living her rich, joyful life for "that kind of nonsense."

Sometimes patients will deny that they have a special road or a special talent that they have suppressed. It should then be pointed out that it is the very fact of the talent's existence, even if it is undiscovered, that has made the patient's life so painful. If there were no such special road, the patient would not feel discontent or tension. As Pascal puts it, "No one is discontented at not being a king except a discrowned king." If the patient were psychologically "fit" for the life he has led, he would have been happy with it. Unhappiness almost invariably indicates the existence of a road not taken, a talent undeveloped, a self not recognized.

The denial of the existence of the third road coincides with an excessive concern for the opinions of others. As Carl Jung, Erik Erikson and others have pointed out, there is a new developmental stage that occurs in adulthood—usually between 35 and 45 years of age—in which the person normally turns from concern with others to the needs of the self. By this time, the adult has defined himself or herself in terms of society; in order to continue growing as a person, there is a fresh need to define the self in terms of more individual, inner-directed concerns. Those who have made this development are not likely to need help. They are with life, for it, part of it. If such people do contract cancer, they usually have the inner resources to fight for their lives on their own. The cancer is likely to grow more slowly, and so can be more readily treated by surgery or other medical means.

Those who develop fast-spreading "terminal" cancers have usually failed to make the change to more inward concerns. To them, the opinions of others still come first; their primary orientation is "other-directed." This neglect of their own inner development seems strongly related to the weakness of their will to live. They suffer from a long-term exhaustion, which stems from investing their emotional energy in ways of expressing and relating that give no inner satisfaction. When such people become ill, they are robbed of even the little support that they have received from outside themselves. In severe illness, one is alone with oneself. The supports of status, prestige, and the opinions of others, diminish considerably in importance. The patient is largely restricted to those psychic supports that come from his inner life—yet it is just those supports that he has neglected. When these patients can be helped to turn their efforts inward, to cultivate the neglected aspects of themselves, the will to live often shows a marked increase in intensity.

In the first chapter, I wrote about Louise, who had spent her entire adult life caring for and largely supporting her husband and children. After the death of her husband, she saw to it that all her children got college educations, but their very success in life, their ability to create independent lives for themselves, eventually

146

left Louise with no role to play in life. In psychotherapy, it developed that she had always enjoyed the ballet. She had very limited financial resources, but still managed to keep up with the activities of the ballet world even though she was seldom able to attend a performance. She would borrow yesterday's newspapers to read reviews, read everything about it she could find in local libraries, and sometimes make trips to the main public library at 42nd Street in New York—an hour's trip each way—to borrow books she could not find elsewhere. Once in a great while, she was able to see a performance. In discussing these rare events, she spoke with real excitement and animation for the first time in therapy. She remembered all the dancers she had ever seen, and talked of each one with expertise. I brought in a professional ballet dancer to talk with her, and she later described this conversation as "one of the best afternoons of my life."

She had never discussed her love for the ballet with her husband or friends; they knew about it, but were not interested themselves and sometimes teased her about it. Such teasing was extremely painful to her, but she had found no way to reply to them except through silence. But during the course of therapy she decided to write a book about the history of ballet in New York City. At first this idea was a very tentative one, and it required a great deal of encouragement to persuade her to actually undertake the project. I went to libraries to get her the books she needed, and later, after I talked with her children, they took on the job of supplying her with research materials. Louise became deeply engrossed in this work. Each day she read and wrote until she was exhausted, slept, and then worked some more. Her whole orientation to life changed. She was excited, fulfilled, enthusiastic. I will never forget visiting Louise in her hospital room, the bed, tables and chairs piled high with library books, with stacks of yellow pads in easy reach. Louise aroused the ire of the nurses because she turned on her light early in the morning and often kept it on long after they felt a hospital patient should be asleep. But I could only be joyful. Louise was making up for a lifetime of lost pleasure. Medical reports indicated that her treatments were proving much more effective, and the growth of the cancer appeared to have stopped.

Unhappily, the weather suddenly turned extremely hot. The hospital was not then air-conditioned, and the rooms and wards reached a temperature that was unbearable for visitors and staff and disastrous for the patients. In a one-week period, a number of patients succumbed to the combination of heat and their illnesses. Louise was one of them. But Louise did not die in despair, consumed by self-contempt. As both she and her children attested, the last months of her life were full of zest and pleasure in life. Even on the day of her death, she was looking to the future. For Louise, as for other patients, it was not a matter of how long she had to live, for she had discovered a self that she could approve; she could be happy on her own terms, not those of others, and for the time that was left to her after she began to work on her book, she lived with an intensity and a joy that she had never known before.

In some cases, a patient's ability to discover the rejected self, or to believe that change is possible, that a third road exists, is hindered by another person. The patient will say, "She (my wife) will never change and I can't leave her because of the children. Every time she makes me feel guilty I know there's no point in going on living." Or, "My father makes me feel like a hopeless failure every time we are together." Or, "Every time my supervisor calls me she makes me realize that I can never succeed at anything." In such situations, a "transaction" is going on that keeps the patient convinced that no change is possible.

Although this type of situation is very painful for the patient, it sometimes offers an excellent therapeutic opportunity for helping him to understand that by a change in his own orientation, he can overcome a seemingly hopeless condition. The patient may be told to sit down with a pencil and paper when he is alone, and to sort out into four or five classes the various methods that the other person uses to make him feel guilty or hopeless. He is then told to number the classes or types and to memorize them according to number. Using this list, the patient tries to predict which method will be used by the other person each time they meet. He says to himself, in effect, "The next time she tries to make me feel guilty, she will use #4 technique."

The efficacy of this procedure is often quite startling. First, it changes the total structure of the situation. The patient is now objectively focused on what is being done, rather than simply reacting to it. We can either observe an object or we can observe our way of looking at it—our response. We cannot do both at the same time. Thus the patient focuses on what is being done rather than on how he feels about it. The patient suddenly finds himself observing—usually in an amused manner—what was previously responded to as a painful assault. No longer does the attack cause the patient to have negative feelings about himself. On the contrary, the knowledge that he has the ability to deal with the attack effectively tends to produce feelings of competence. He learns that no matter what the outside situation is, the important thing is his response to it, and that this response *can* change.

There is also a secondary gain. The disruption of the transaction is unconsciously perceived by the other person. Since the transaction is no longer "working," it is usually abandoned, and the techniques that tended to mobilize the patient's feelings of guilt or inadequacy cease.

Susan, for instance, who was a teacher in a small school, had a superior who constantly denigrated her work. The superior was a black, while Susan was white, and racial resentments seemed to be part of the superior's motivation. But even though she recognized this fact, Susan's long-standing feelings that everything she did spontaneously, as herself, would bring her rejection and attack were reinforced each time she was criticized.

After Susan started to use the "prediction game" technique she found that the criticisms no longer bothered her. She was able to make an objective evaluation as to whether or not they were valid. Inside of a month, the criticisms had stopped, and an excellent relationship with her superior developed, lasting for three years until Susan married and moved away. The transaction having been refused, Susan and her superior found that they really liked each other, and became friends as well as colleagues.

The patient's turning from concern with the opinions and reactions of others to concern with the needs and growth of the self is often marked by a crisis. This existential crisis—or existential opportunity—usually occurs after a patient has truly begun to understand that there is a possible third road. The crisis usually begins with the patient feeling as though all his drives and needs were markedly intensified—as if there were a sort of emotional typhoon raging within him. His past techniques for relating to others have become weakened with the realization that they are self-defeating; but he has not yet attained full confidence in his new ways of relating. There is thus a sense of being lost, of drifting without an anchor.

Often the first sign of the onset of this crisis will be a special request on the part of the patient. Patients who have been considerate, even overly considerate of my time and other activities, will suddenly ask for a special appointment on a Saturday or holiday. My wife has come to expect, over the years, that I will be absent for a few hours on any Thanksgiving or Christmas Eve. I try to view such requests in the context of the particular patient's progress and needs. The patient seems to be making a final test of the validity of my caring—which is, after all, the patient's "lifeline"—before making the leap out of the safety of his life-long ways of living. If it is humanly possible, I fulfill such requests on the terms they are made. I do *not*, however, analyze or explain it to the patient until long after the crisis is over.

In my experience, the fulfillment of such a request will not bring other such requests, or cause a future lack of consideration for the therapist. The patient will feel that this one test is enough—if the therapist responds to the testing with understanding, without resentment, and treats the request as though it were perfectly valid, which it is.

Although the concept of the existential crisis is a fairly new one in psychotherapy, it has long been described in literature and myth. The concept of the "final battle" between life and death, expansion and contraction, being and non-being, is found in many cultures throughout history. Such myths foretell that things will get worse before the final confrontation—the appearance of the Antichrist in Christian theology is one example—and that there will be a period of great tension and confusion before the final choice is made between light and darkness.

In certain therapeutic situations, it is possible to speed up the resolution of this crisis by sending the patient off alone somewhere—where he will have no accustomed roles to play and where neither he nor anyone else has any expectations as to how he will behave. The absence of accustomed roles permits his inner resources of wish and desire to come closer to consciousness. As one patient put it, the person "lets his feet take him where they will." The patient observes what he does and whether or not he enjoys it. In a sense, the patient is asking himself: "Will the real John Doe please stand up."

The patient should understand in advance that this is a learning and growing situation and not a vacation. He should be warned that the first several days he may be depressed and anxious, but beyond that he "plays it by ear." With a full grasp of what is being attempted, patients often make very real progress during such periods. The timing of such a venture is somewhat delicate, however. It should be undertaken only after a full encounter with the therapist has been achieved and the philosophy of the search is competely clear. Goethe wrote that "a talent grows best in solitude; character is perfected in the stream of the world." But these patients have *too much* "character." They have lived in the stream of the world too completely. And they have neglected developing "that one talent which it is death to hide"—their fundamental creativity—and it is this neglect that is killing them.

A great many therapeutic situations do not, of course, permit the usage of this procedure. The patient may be too ill to leave the hospital, or lack the financial re-

153

sources to go off alone. But other arrangements are sometimes possible. A patient may be able to take one day a week, in his own city, to do just as he or she pleases, without planned activities. Anne, for instance, who was a housewife, decided to take Wednesdays as "my own day." She was able to arrange for baby-sitters for these Wednesdays, and from nine to four she was "free." She would drive into the city from her suburban home and do what she wished. In spite of being on crutches because of a leg amputation, she found herself going to theaters and museums, sitting in the park looking at trees and water and people romping with their dogs, wandering in stores, or having lunch either by herself or with old friends. In Anne's case, a full existential crisis was not precipitated, but there was a remarkable loosening of her previously tight defenses. She developed a growing sense that she herself deserved at least as much caring as did her children and husband.

As a secondary gain, her friends told her how much they envied and respected her for taking a day to be hers alone. Several other suburban women subsequently asked if they could accompany her. For the last year of her life, she knew that she was liked and respected by many people, and she no longer felt like the deviant, outcast failure she had always conceived herself to be.

When there is anxiety on the part of a spouse—or the patient—that a time of separation during which the patient goes off alone may lead to a permanent loss of the marital relationship, it can sometimes be eased by reference to Arnold Toynbee's concept of "withdrawal and return." This concept embodies the idea that it is sometimes necessary for a person or a society to withdraw from a problem in order to gather and reorganize his forces before returning with greater strength and coherence to deal with it. In this connection, it is interesting that the word "convalescence" derives from the name for the ancient Roman bugle call that signaled the troops to break off fighting, withdrawing *in order to reorganize before returning to battle.* To fight for one's life against cancer, a similar re-ordering of one's emotional forces is often vital to the will to survive.

The techniques described in this chapter were used to varying degrees and in differing combinations with my terminal cancer patients. Each patient had his or her particular areas of difficulty in taking the first steps along the third road toward a renewed sense of self and the ability to fight for one's life that goes with it. For some, the most difficult step was to rediscover that secret dream for themselves that they had long ago abandoned or repressed: their particular talents had often been so completely disavowed that it was as though they had never existed. Others still cherished some special ambition, but regarded the achievement of it as beyond hope. Still others were trapped like a fly in the web of other people's demands and opinions: in whatever direction they tried to move they found themselves confronted by a different strand of the web that they had allowed and unconsciously trained other people to weave about them.

Take the case of Linda, for example. As a teenager, Linda had wanted to go to college. She wanted a career for herself. Her parents, however, were horrified by the idea. They believed that a career was out of the question for a nice girl from a good family. Trying desperately to please her parents, Linda married the man they approved of and had four children. Her husband was wealthy, and from the outside it might have appeared that she had a contented and fortunate life. In actuality, her marriage had been an unhappy one for many years. The expectation that she should be content was to her a dreadful trap. She derived no fulfillment from her role as wife and mother, but felt imprisoned, seeing her life as one of never-ending servitude to others. Out of desperation, she became involved with another man— one who encouraged her to lead her own life. But once again, her parents, together with her husband, persuaded her that she was wrong, and that she would destroy the lives of her children. They took the attitude that her affair—her attempt to become herself—was an illness. She gave up her relationship with the other man, and allowed herself to be enfolded once again within the claustrophobic arms of her "forgiving" family. Four months later, she noticed a lump in her breast.

Linda had a mastectomy and then a hysterectomy for the spreading cancer. But then she was told that there was no further operation that could help; the cancer was permeating her body, and was beyond treatment. Shortly after she was told that her cancer was terminal, Linda came to me. In Linda's case, it seemed particularly important that she spend some time outside the confines of her family situation. I encouraged her to work part time in a department store, and to use the money she earned to attend college classes two or three nights a week. Her husband and parents were furious, of course. It was, however, my job to be her ally, to assure her that she should and must do what *she* wanted to do. This was a situation in which the very fact of her cancer being terminal seemed to give her strength to stand up to her family. Since she expected to die, the opposition of her husband and parents had less effect than it had previously. And she knew that I was with her all the way.

She persisted, working and studying until her youngest child entered high school. At that point, despite terrible guilt feelings, she became a full-time student and began divorce proceedings. The pleasure and satisfaction she took from her new life were by now strong enough so that she was able to withstand the outrage and the tearful entreaties of her family.

Today Linda is a college librarian. Every summer she travels in Europe and she has never felt better in her life. She is presently involved with a man she had loved since high school, but whom she had never been allowed to date because he was "the wrong religion." For now, though, she doesn't want to remarry. The freedom of choice she has gained is still too new for her—and too

157

precious—to be easily relinquished. She has been able to help her children to understand why she had to leave their father. Having discovered who she really is, she is able to communicate that self and her needs to others. As she puts it, "They love me in spite of the fact that they think I'm some kind of nut."

This last statement of Linda's tells, in a way, the whole story. She has found the third road. Previously, she had believed that she could be loved only by denying her true self. That was one road, and a destructive one. The only other road that she could conceive of was to be herself, but to lose the love of others in the process. Now, she recognizes that she can be her own "kind of nut" and still retain the love of other people. True, she lost the love of her husband—but she had long since stopped loving him. His love was so thin that he loved her only so long as she lived up to his expectations. Each of us may seem "some kind of nut" to some of the people we care about—but if they truly care about us, they will love us even so. If they do not truly care, then surely they are not worth destroying ourselves for, no matter what our relationship to them may be.

Another of my patients, Stanley, made some surprising (to him) discoveries about the reactions of other people once he learned to be himself. Stanley's father had died when he was six. In common with all children in the face of such an event, Stanley felt that his father's death would not have occurred if he himself had been a better boy. Feeling that he must change so that his mother would not also abandon him, Stanley became a quiet, serious boy. He made excellent grades and went through college and graduate school on scholarships. Becoming a very successful and very well-liked professional, he wrote several books that sold widely in their field. Yet these successes were, as he put it, "like ashes in my mouth." Nothing gave him any real pleasure or satisfaction except the time he spent building model ships, a hobby he had enjoyed since childhood. Otherwise he existed like a robot, consumed by feelings of emptiness.

A terminal cancer patient, Stanley came to me for help. At this point he was almost totally lacking in a sense of self. When I suggested, after two months of therapy, that he go off by himself for a while, in order to try to be concerned with his own needs, he simply could not comprehend what I meant. If he and his wife were to take separate vacations, he said, "I wouldn't know what to do with myself. Unless I talked it over with her, how would I know what I enjoyed doing that day? I'd just sit there." He needed somebody else to tell him what he had enjoyed!

Very gradually, through the use of the "time machine" technique and other methods, I was able to help Stanley to understand how and why he had given his selfhood away as a child, in reaction to his father's death. He began to realize why his successes meant nothing to him —they had not been achieved *for himself*, but simply out of the fear that if he was not a good boy and a successful man, he would be abandoned. Yet, in the process, he had abandoned himself. Because he had no true self, he did not relate to other people in a "real" way; the fact that he was universally liked also meant nothing to him, for he recognized that what people liked was merely a façade. He never caused other people any offense because he had no true self to either express or defend.

After about six months of therapy, his cancer began to slow in its growth, and to become quiescent. This medical change coincided with a change in his way of looking at himself. He gradually began to see that he had a right to be himself. His behavior toward others became more "real"; it now included two people, the other person *and* himself, whereas it had previously been based only upon the requirements of the other person. To his great surprise, his professional success increased. He knew that he was no longer universally liked. But he discovered that the people he really cared about liked him *more,* even though others did not like him as much and some not at all. For the first time in his life he began to enjoy the friendship of others. Even more important, he discovered that he could be friends with *himself,* could enjoy his *own* company. Being alone, he found, could also be richly rewarding, now that he had a self to be alone with.

For the past several years, Stanley's cancer has remained quiescent, although it remains present in x-rays. Stanley now truly enjoys his work, takes pleasure in his success and in his social life. Like Linda, he found that a third road did in fact exist. Because he likes his life, he has developed the strength to fight for it. His terminal cancer developed when he was dead inside—emtpy of feeling and devoid of self. Now that he is himself, and expresses that self, he is alive inside, and it is the cancer that is quiescent.

The World of the Cancer Patient 9

As has been indicated throughout this book, the world of the terminal cancer patient is a special one, both physically and psychologically. The psychological life history of the cancer patient sets him apart from the individuals that a therapist would see in a usual big city practice. He cannot be helped by traditional therapeutic approaches; new methods, such as those of crisis psychotherapy, are necessary to free the patient from the narrow world in which he has been trapped, to restore his ability to fight for his life.

In addition to his particular psychological problems,

the cancer patient also must often deal with chronic pain. The amount of published material on the situation of the patient in chronic pain is surprisingly small. In one of the few serious works on the subject, Buytend- jick has commented, "Modern man regards pain merely as an unpleasant fact which, like every other evil, he must do his best to get rid of. To do this, it is generally held, there is no need for any reflection on the phe- nomena itself." Yet, to help the patient regain his will to live, this aspect of his special world must also be fully understood.

The universe of the patient in chronic pain bears considerable similarity to the nightmare. There are three basic structural components to the terror dream: (1) Terrible things are being done to us and worse are threatened; (2) Outside forces are in control, and our will is helpless; (3) There is no set time-limit, and we cannot predict when it will be over. The person in chronic pain is in the same basic situation. To under- stand that the cancer patient lives in a waking night- mare, and to communicate this understanding to the patient, can often help the patient to withstand the assault of his pain.

Our understanding of pain is usually based upon acute transitory pain—the toothache, the burn, the cut or bruise. This type of pain is conducted very rapidly through the nervous system, causes defensive reflexes to be brought into play, and usually passes relatively quickly. We are taught from childhood to regard such pain as a good and useful warning. When faced with chronic pain, the individual tends to generalize from his experience with acute transitory pain. This generalization leaves much to be desired; indeed, its validity is questionable. To regard chronic pain as a "warning" confuses the problem. For it does not tell us what to do, and there are no defensive reflexes with which we can react to it. It continues long after we have put ourselves in the care of a physician. It does not help us to act, and may be so severe as to disrupt potentially useful activities and habits. Chronic pain is simply a state of existence.

Chronic pain thus comes to seem both inexplicable and meaningless. Mental suffering seems to follow naturally from our thoughts and actions; it reflects our view of ourself. But chronic physical pain is alien. It does not appear to follow from what we are or have done. It appears to be meaningless; but since it is very difficult to accept real experience as unreasonable, we attempt to give it meaning. Our ancient guilts and anxieties are aroused, and we try to assign the pain to these insufficient causes. Every great religion and philosophy has tried to explore the meaning of pain, but in our own anti-metaphysical society it is largely ignored. It is something we would like to shut our eyes to—and thus, when it must be borne, we have no traditional ways of dealing with it.

As human beings, we normally try to interact with our environment. But we cannot interact with pain; we can only bear it. "It is a peculiarity of man," says

Victor Frankl, "that he can live only by looking to the future . . ." But with chronic pain there is a real loss of time perspective—we are bound to the immediate *now* of the pain itself. A further aspect of the problem is that chronic pain is experienced in isolation. The French author Alphonse Daudet said, "Pain is always something new for him who suffers, but banal to those about him. They will all get used to it except myself."

The loud loneliness of pain thus presses us toward a psychic regression. Our dignity and hard-won adult status is weakened. Our body image becomes blurred; the pain seems to obliterate the rest of the physical self. We are conscious only of the area that is producing such overwhelming sensations. From the complex adult perception of the body, we are thrown back upon a more childlike body-image. This loss of our adult sense of ourselves is further aggravated by the fact that—as in childhood—we have to depend upon others to take many of the important actions in our lives.

With the cancer patient, the degree of pain experienced often seems to be connected with how the person feels about his or her life as a whole. As Gotthard Booth has pointed out, ". . . pain is frequently more dependent on the morale than on the physical condition of the patient." This phenomenon is known to everyone in other situations—as for instance, the football player who does not feel the pain of his bone fracture, and continues in the game. There can be no pain without the involvement of the higher nervous centers, and it is how these centers handle, absorb and integrate the pain that determines the individual's perception of it and his ability to resist it.

A fascinating portrait of the cancer patient's reaction to pain is given in Tolstoi's *The Death of Ivan Illytch.* In fact, this novella, written almost a hundred years ago, portrays with uncanny exactitude and extraordinary insight a life history that conforms in almost every way to the profile of the cancer-prone personality presented here. Tolstoi's novella is one of the frequent examples of the artist "getting there first," far ahead of the scientist. In *The Death of Ivan Illytch,* it is only when Ivan realizes the total meaninglessness of his life that he is overwhelmed by the pain of cancer. As long as there seems to him to be a valid meaning to his existence, he is able to resist the pain and retain both control and dignity.

A woman of my acquaintance who had had terribly severe pain for many years, resulting from an inner ear disorder, nevertheless continued her active, useful and ebullient life. When asked how she did it, she responded, "When the pain is severe, I rise above it and look at it from a higher level." This explanation should not be dismissed merely as "hysteroid." Because she was able to retain control over herself and the pain she was experiencing, she was not overwhelmed by it.

Generally, as cancer patients begin to rediscover their previously rejected true selves, and to find a meaning to their lives, they are better able to handle their pain. As one woman, who was making considerable progress in therapy, said, "It's like the difference between child-birth and other pains. In labor, you know that some-thing will be produced at the end. It's never as bad as when the pain doesn't produce anything."

In helping the cancer patient to deal with his or her pain, the approach must once again be focused on the specific individual. There can be no rules as to how this is done, only a recognition of its importance. Each patient must be helped to find the answer most natural to him, to his own sense of meaning, not the meaning that makes sense to the therapist. Some patients may be able to make sense of their pain in terms of the fresh understanding of themselves that has grown out of their cancer. "Your pain," says Kahlil Gibran in *The Prophet*, "is the breaking of the shell that encloses your under-standing." For patients who have always resisted facing their true selves, who have always feared that they would not be loved if they revealed that self, there can be meaning in the idea that their cancer has brought them to the point where they must embrace themselves or die. To discover that they can be loved as themselves makes the pain acceptable to them, and with their new strength they find themselves able to resist it.

Other patients may come to grips with their pain in other ways. Recognizing that the experience of their cancer can never be taken from them, that after it is over they will never need to fear anything again, they may feel, in Nietzsche's words, "That which does not kill me, makes me stronger." Still others may see the pain they have as *existing in itself*; the fact of *their* experiencing it is thus viewed as saving someone else from the experience. The effectiveness of the psychotherapist thus depends, in large part, on his ingenuity in helping the patient find his own best answer. As the will to live reasserts itself, many patients come to feel, in the dark and wise words of Dostoevski, that "There is only one thing I dread; not to be worthy of my sufferings."

When pain is unusually severe or unusually resistant, it should be asked whether there is a purpose behind the pain in the case of the particular patient. Does it hold off guilt? Does it provide him with a sense of being "real" that he desperately needs. Is there a message in his pain? Severe pain can, for instance, be a substitute for overwhelming mental anguish. In the medical literature there are cases in which chronic pain has been relieved by drugs or other means, only to be followed immediately by the emotional breakdown or suicide of the patient. Yet our cultural orientation toward pain—that it is evil and must be immediately relieved—is so strong that the possibility that the patient is telling us something through his pain is often ignored.

In cancer patients, especially, the therapist must be on guard in situations where pain is unusually severe. The typical patient with terminal cancer has, after all, been living with great mental anguish for many years prior to the development of the malignancy. The possibility exists that the cancer developed not only because the individual's resistance was low—because all his psychic energy was invested in protecting himself against his mental anguish—but also that the cancer is in some way a physical substitute for unbearable mental suffering. Although this is a conjectural point, it is important to recognize it as a possible reality. And in such cases, the psychic suffering must be relieved before the patient can safely be deprived of the physical pain that—to him—is easier to bear than the despair he has lived with for so long.

Regardless of how the pain is perceived by the individual patient, pity for the person in pain is extremely corrosive. When the patient perceives that he or she is being pitied, it weakens the ability to deal with the situation. Pity reinforces the patient's feeling of helplessness because it is an indication of a lower status. The patient's strivings to retain dignity and adulthood can be helped through empathy, emotional contact and respect. Pity only weakens the patient's will to live, and this fact must not only be understood by the therapist but also communicated to the patient's family. For this and other reasons, it is essential that contact between the family and the therapist be initiated and maintained.

Since the patient usually lives in—and is a part of— a total family situation, successful therapy must take into account this aspect of the world of the cancer patient. Traditional therapeutic doctrine insists that contact with the family should be kept to the minimum, but this maxim cannot be followed in crisis therapy. With honesty and a full open encounter between patient and therapist, there is no need for the therapist to fear that the patient will feel contact with the family to be an act of "disloyalty." Furthermore, the issues at stake are too large—literally a matter of life and death—for either patient or therapist to be concerned with general rules or customs.

In a profound sense, the patient's family defines his life-space. It is a part of his reality, and cannot be ignored. As Stanley, who had previously undergone traditional therapy put it, "Reality does so exist!" Thus the therapist who deals with terminal cancer patients must take this reality into full account.

The therapist gets to know the spouse—and/or children—for several important reasons. To begin with, the information acquired from the family might not arise in sessions with the patient himself for quite a long time. And if the patient's will to live is to be revived, it must be done quickly—time is not something that can be taken for granted in crisis therapy. Time must be measured in weeks and months, not in years.

Secondly, it is important to reduce the pressure on the patient as much as possible. There are several types of family pressure that often have a strong influence on the cancer patient. To begin with, the patient is aware that he is expected to remain the same person he always was in family interactions. By helping the family understand that the patient must *change* in order to be able to fight for his life, and that such growth does not mean the loss of the relationship, but generally its strengthening, much unconscious pressure can be eased. When a spouse has inordinate fears concerning the possibility of such change, it is important to know that fact; it can often lead to a deeper understanding of the patient's problem areas.

With terminal cancer patients, the family often accepts the medical opinion that the situation is hopeless and that the patient cannot possibly survive for more than a few months. As has been shown in several case histories throughout this book, *remissions do take place,* regardless of medical opinion, when the patient is sufficiently motivated to fight for his life and brings all his resources to that fight. But even if the patient cannot be "cured," even if he is unable to fight the cancer to a standstill, it is still possible for him to enjoy the last months or years of his life in a new affirmative way, looking to the future and at home with his true self. This alone is a goal worth fighting for in the most tenacious way.

But when the family assumes that the patient will die, that there is no hope, it becomes harder than ever for the patient to hope and to fight for his life. For the family to give up is often, of course, a self-protective measure. It immunizes the family to some extent from involvement in the patient's suffering—family members are able to tell themselves, "Well, it will soon be over." Yet such an attitude is quickly communicated to the patient, and it has a profoundly depressing effect. If others will not hope for him, why should he hope for himself? In addition, it serves to confirm the patient's conviction that he is unlovable.

I have on several occasions found it necessary to say

171

to the family of a cancer patient, "Let's face something." This phrase has very strong negative connotations. It leads the family to expect that I am going to say, "Joe is dying." Thus, when I say instead, "Joe is *alive*," the family members experience a profound shock, a shock that often succeeds in jolting them into the realization that *they* have already considered Joe dead.

These reminders are also necessary to prevent the family from infantilizing the patient, thus robbing him of the strength he needs to grow and develop. There is a marked tendency in our culture to wrap the patient in a kind of psychological cotton padding—to make him into a helpless child. This kind of attitude must be avoided. The family should be helped to understand that "rest" is not a particularly useful medication, and the patient should *not* be prevented from action. There are illnesses, such as tuberculosis and hepatitis, in which activity should be limited for medical reasons, but cancer is not one of them. The patient should be encouraged to be as active as possible, stopping just short of getting "falling-down exhausted." Frequently, both the family and the physician go on the assumption that the patient's activity level should be kept as low as possible, and thereby hinder him in his attempt to find and express his own path and way of being. I have often found it necessary to take a strong stand against this tendency.

Another reason for establishing a relationship with the family is to help them with realistic planning. Real problems do exist on many levels, from financial difficulties to techniques of mourning, and these should be discussed where necessary. In itself, such a discussion often reduces the psychological load on the patient, particularly when he or she has been the primary bread-winner.

The therapist should also be concerned with preparing children for the possibility of a parent's death, so that the sons or daughters do not come to feel that "If I was a better boy or girl, mother would not have left me." This emotional burden, as we have seen, is the kind that in itself can dispose a person to the fear of relationships and the self-contempt that are an integral part of the cancer-prone personality. The possibility should be considered, in fact, that the recurrence of cancer in several generations of the same family has more to do with this constantly reinforced emotional burden than it does with genetics as such.

Parents should be taught how to deal with the preparation of children for the possibility of a patient's death. On some occasions, however, it may be necessary for the therapist to undertake this important task himself. One patient of mine was bedridden at home, and I went to see her twice a week. She and her husband had a ten-year-old son, with whom the father found himself unable to discuss his wife's illness. Frequently, after a session with the mother, I would walk to my car with the boy, and we would talk for half an hour or so about his feelings. I explained to him, again and again, that we do not know what causes cancer, but we *do* know that it is *not* caused by the behavior of others. It was not a matter of who the boy was or how he behaved. The cancer would have come anyway. His mother loved him very much, and was fighting hard to get well, but even if she did not, there was no way in which it could be considered his fault.*

Often, it is necessary to continue to see members of the family—children and/or a surviving spouse—for a considerable time if a patient does succumb to the disease. This work to prevent the fact of the loved one's death from doing more emotional damage than absolutely inevitable, is simply a part of the therapist's job. Patients will frequently request such help, and it cannot be refused. If it is not requested, it should be offered. Often there is no money for the family to pay for visits of this kind, a fact which any therapist working with the terminally ill must accept beforehand.

The loss of real communication between the terminally ill person and those closest to the patient is an extremely common event. Family members may try to quiet the patient's fears by avoiding any discussion whatever of his illness. If the subject is broached at all, there is usually an attempt to pretend that the patient will get well. As we have seen, there are cases in which the patient has had a remission. But, having been told by the physician that there is no hope, family members usually do not really accept that possibility. When they do talk about the possibility of recovery, they are saying something that they do not themselves believe, and the patient inevitably senses that fact. For the patient, this

---

* An extremely useful book in this area is *Learning to Say Goodbye: When a Parent Dies,* by Eda LeShan (Macmillan, 1976).

is an extremely stressful situation, increasing his sense of loneliness. It breaks his life-lines to others—life-lines that must be based upon honesty. It increases the patient's fears. Thus, the therapist should make every effort to see that the patient has as many open and honest channels for relating as possible.

The importance of honesty not only between the therapist and patient, but also between family members and the patient is perhaps best illustrated by the following case history. George, a 67-year-old man with an abdominal cancer, was confined to a hospital bed. He knew that he had a fatal cancer, but had not told his wife, Anna, that he knew this to be so—in order to "spare" her. He kept up a front of unworried good spirits. Yet, in actuality, Anna did know that her husband was dying. She hid *this* knowledge from George, insisting that the "doctors said he would be all right." These two people had been married 42 years. They loved and cared deeply for one another, but were unable to talk together about the most important thing in the world for each of them. Since neither of them dared to let this subject come up, there were progessively more and more things they could not talk about, because they might lead to the forbidden subject of George's likely death. Needing each other more now than at any other time of their lives, George and Anna were each cut off from the one person who could help most—the other. Anna spent a great deal of time at the hospital, but although they were physically close, there was an emotional wall between them, and it was growing higher all the time.

You Can Fight for Your Life

Both Anna and George had told me of their unwillingness to admit what they knew to the other. I felt that this was an intolerable situation, one that was hurting them both, and I decided to do something about it. Without warning them in advance, and with much anxiety, I went into George's hospital room one afternoon when Anna was there, and said, "It's time for you two to really talk to each other about what's happening. As you both know, the illness is cancer, and it's serious. We are all very frightened and there is something to be frightened about. But nobody is giving up hope. We are going to fight this thing. There are a lot more tools we can use, and if we should run out of those, new ones are being discovered all the time. No one is giving up. We are going to try to win and we have a good fighting chance. But it's dangerous and frightening and sad, and some things are worth some tears. I know how each of you feels, and it's time for you to let each other know. You've loved and helped each other all your lives, and you need each other now."

This is a dramatic example, but the need for action of this sort is frequent in hospitals. Anyone who has ever dealt with terminally ill patients of any kind would recognize it immediately. The same need can exist outside of a hospital situation, of course. In other circumstances, the rapprochement between George and Anna might have been effected by having an individual session with each of them, and letting them open communication in their own way. It could have taken place

176

at my office, or at a patient's home. Whatever the location, however, I always leave the room afterwards, but remain where I can be reached if questions arise that I may be able to answer.

Unhappily, physicians and nurses often encourage such deceptions between family members as existed with George and Anna. The difficulty is that both physicians and nurses also tend to think of the patient as "all but dead." From their viewpoint, terminal cancer means death, and nothing else. They too must be shocked into recognition that the patient is still alive. With physicians, this can be a particular problem. My work is almost bound to be resented on some level. The physician has said, "There is nothing more I can do." The fact that I believe there is much to be done, that even the terminal patient can be helped in ways that will at least allow him to discover his true self before he dies, and, at best, restore to him the will to live, the belief in himself that will help him fight for his life, inevitably causes the physician mixed feelings. It is not that they are uncaring, of course, but simply that their perception of cancer as a disease rests on narrow assumptions that have for too long been widely held.

With nurses, the problem is somewhat different. I once carried out a test at a hospital, to see how long it took the nurses to answer the call bells from rooms of various patients. Statistically, it took them longer to answer a call from a room in which the patient was near death than one in which the patient was not. This is an entirely natural reaction. Nurses are often under great strain, and there is a limit to their resources just as there is to mine or anyone else's. Yet, the fact remains that the cancer patient is profoundly aware of the fact that it takes the nurses a long time to come to them. This can easily be taken as one more form of rejection, confirming their doubts about their own worth. When I made my tests at the hospital, the nurses were called together afterward, and they were informed of the results. At first they hotly denied that they delayed in getting to the rooms of dying patients. But the time charts were irrefutable. After I had explained why these delays were of such concern to me, the nurses responded by entering into a very open and often emotional discussion. They talked about their pain and anguish at the frequent deaths and that the more they knew the patient as a person, the greater their suffering. Afterwards, a number of them told me that it had been a very good session, and that it had made them aware of how much their presence really did mean.

The world of the cancer patient, in spite of its pain and sadness, can lead back into the world of the living— even for those whose cases are regarded as hopeless. The therapist must not hold out *false* hope. But, on the other hand, it is my own conviction that the word "hopeless" should be banished from the world of the cancer patient. My job as a therapist is to help the patient banish it.

What It Means to Fight for One's Life 10

My purpose in writing this book has not been to prove or disprove anything. We are a long way from solving the mysteries of cancer, in all its complexities. I have tried to describe a profoundly important element—one aspect of the study of cancer that has been seriously neglected, and to report as carefully as I could on what seem to me to be dramatic and essential leads in understanding this disease. Beyond that, I am concerned about those individuals, who, after reading this book, suspect they may have "cancer-prone personalities" as well as those who have cancer and want to use every possible resource for recovery.

Some readers have probably found themselves identifying with the life pattern of the cancer patients described. It is important to remember that I have been talking about *a constellation* of factors. Any particular symptom, in isolation, has no special significance. Equally important, I have been describing people with a *life history*, not a temporary period of difficulty. All of us have periods of suffering, frustration, despair, sorrow, loneliness, loss; all of us are not going to develop cancer.

For those who find themselves responding as if the book is a warning—a message to be taken personally and seriously—this need not be an experience in terror, but an important opportunity for self-examination.

Thousands of women were grateful to Mrs. Ford and Mrs. Rockefeller when they talked openly and frankly about breast cancer; their candor undoubtedly saved many lives as women became acutely conscious and concerned about self-examination and medical guidance. I would hope that this book might encourage a different kind of self-examination—a search for one's unique authenticity as a human being.

There are some basic and legitimate questions we can raise with ourselves—and if our answers surprise or shock us, it may well be time to examine our life. In addition to medical checkups, here is a list of appropriate questions one might ask oneself, related to those emotional states that seem so often to be significant in the development of some malignancies:

1. Am I able to express anger when I feel it most strongly?
2. Do I try to make the best of things, no matter what happens, without ever complaining?
3. Do I have a variety of interests and pleasures in life, or, are all my energies focused on one relationship (to work, or spouse, or child, etc.) so that if I lost that relationship, I would no longer have any reason to live? (For example, if I have to retire, would I just as well die? Or when the children are gone, will I still feel my life is worth living?)
4. Do I think of myself as a lovable, worthwhile person, or have I felt worthless much of the time? Do I often feel lonely, rejected, isolated from others?
5. Am I doing what I want to do with my life? Are my relationships satisfying? Do I feel reasonably optimistic or quite hopeless about ever fulfilling myself?
6. If I were told right now that I had only six months to live, would I go on doing what I am doing right now? Or do I have secret unfulfilled dreams, ambitions, desires of which I am ashamed, and which have plagued me all my life?

7. If I were told I had a terminal illness, would I experience some sense of relief?

If such questions do bring a sense of shock it need not be a time for despair and hopelessness but an opportunity for taking charge of one's life—beginning to search out needed alternatives and finding the courage to change those things that block the realization of one's own unique potential. The most important thing to keep in mind is this: *it is possible to be concerned and responsible towards others without sacrificing one's own life.*

So many people are writing so many books on "realizing one's full potential" that it may seem anticlimatic that after dramatically claiming emotions can sometimes cause cancer, I seem to be recommending preventive procedures that sound superficial—over-popularized generalities.

As a matter of fact, when such ideas are presented seriously, without the promise of quick or easy solutions, they may very well *have* an influence on the cancer statistics! In any event, since the person with a cancer-prone personality frequently does deny his individuality, it is inevitable to think of the personal search for self-hood as a possibly preventive measure.

This would apply equally to the person who now has cancer. If one is being treated by surgery, radiation or chemotherapy, the likelihood of recovery is far greater if one is also taking into consideration one's emotional well-being. (Recently Dr. Carl Simonton has shown that the therapeutic effects of radiation for cancer patients can often be markedly increased if radiation therapy is combined with a special form of meditation he is using.)

In one such case, a woman consulted a psychiatrist when she learned that her malignancy was so far advanced she could not expect to live for more than a year. She wanted help in facing her approaching death. The psychiatrist asked if there was anything she had always dreamed of doing, and the woman, who was widowed and childless, said she had always wanted to take a trip around the world. The psychiatrist suggested that since she was still ambulatory and might be for a while, there was no reason why she should not take all her money and invest it in such a trip; after all, if she was going to die within a year, what was she saving it for? The woman took the longest and most luxurious trip she could find. Her health began to improve remarkably in the course of the trip. She returned, went for a medical checkup and was told by her doctor that the cancer was apparently "in total remission." The psychiatrist reported, "She was now practically penniless and furious at me for getting her into such a fix! But we soon found her a job and now she travels whenever she can. I keep getting postcards from all over the world—it's been going on now for about ten years!"

I do not mean to suggest that there are always—or even often—such happy endings, but even if the lady had eventually died, in what style she would have made her last exit! What she did was to say to herself, *"My life matters to me,"* and when we do that, we may be beginning the most important part of our lives, however brief the time may be.

A patient told me, "I know that I'm intelligent, I have courage, and my opinions are as good as anyone else's. Just knowing this has made a big difference in my whole life. I can see the good things I've given my children, not just the bad things. I think I even love them and my husband a lot more now." Another patient said, "You know, Doc, for the first time in my life, I like myself. I'm not half so bad a guy as I always felt I was." A brilliant woman with special skills in theoretical research had been blocked completely for nine years in her ability to do work in her field and was filled with self-doubt and self-dislike. One day she said with triumph and joy, "I started work on an article last night. I have it mapped out and the first two pages written. I think it's going to be pretty good." A 39-year-old woman who had never had a love relationship told me one Monday morning of her wonderful weekend at the beach with a man she had met six months previously. As they had watched the sun go down, she had felt inside like the colors of the sunset. The affair begun that night was one of deep meaning to both of them, and she was able to give and receive the kind of love she had never known existed. Each one of these patients was dying from cancer. None of them lived more than one year after the reported incident. All of them lived "fuller lives" than some people who live into their 90's.

Cancer often kills. Yet there seem to be times when getting cancer can become the beginning of living. The search for one's own being, the discovery of the life one needs to live, can be one of the strongest weapons against disease.

There are, still, of course, many mysteries surrounding cancer. There is no way to predict—no known time-table—for when these mysteries will be solved. But we are beginning to understand that no disease state of any kind can ever be considered "entirely physical"; that every aspect of the human person is involved in all dimensions of sickness and health. From this vantage point, surgery, radiation, drug therapies, prevention of environmental hazards are not enough, by themselves. There is much more to it.

Several years ago, walking along a city street, I saw a familiar face in the crowd, moving towards me. It was the face of a woman patient I had not seen or heard from for over a year. She had had a terminal malignancy and we had worked together in psychotherapy for about five years. When she first came to see me, therapy was the court of last resort; her doctor, the specialists she had consulted, could offer her no alternative treatment.

After she felt she wanted to terminate therapy she still kept in touch with me from time to time. Then her calls stopped altogether, and while at times I had wondered how she was doing—and even worried about her silence—I had not yet felt I should intrude on her life if she did not wish to see me.

She was walking so quickly, with such a light but determined stride, that she almost passed by before she noticed me. She smiled happily, hugged me briefly and then with a wave of her hand as she went on her way, said she was in a hurry, and shouted back at me, "I've been too busy *living* to get in touch with you!"

I watched her as she disappeared again. Going somewhere important; on her way. Alive. Living.

Selected Bibliography of Research Studies on the Relationship Between Psychological Factors and Cancer

General Overviews, Symposia, and Surveys of the Field

ACHTERBERG, J., SIMONTON, O. C., and MATTHEWS-SIMONTON, S., *Stress, Psychological Factors, and Cancer.* Fort Worth, Texas, New Medicine Press, 1976.

Annals of New York Academy of Sciences. Conference on Psychological Aspects of Cancer. Vol. 125, 1966.

Annals of New York Academy of Sciences, Second Conference on Psychological Aspects of Cancer. Vol. 164, 1968.

BALTRUSCH, H. J. F. "Psychosomatic Cancer Research: Present Status and Future Perspectives." In *Psychologie et Cancer.* Paris, Masson, 1978.

———, "Psychotherapy with Cancer Patients." In *Therapy in Psychosomatic Medicine,* edited by F. Antonelli. Rome, Pozzi, 1977.

———, "Results of Clinical Psychosomatic Cancer Research." *Psychosomatic Medicine,* Vol. 5, 175–208, 1975.

BROWN, J. H., VARSAMIS, M. B., TOEWS, J., and SHANE, M., "Psychology and Oncology: A Review." *Canadian Journal of Psychiatry,* Vol. 192, 219-222, 1974.

GENGERELLI, J. A. and KIRKNER, F. J. (eds.), *The Psychological Variables in Human Cancer.* Berkeley, University of California Press, 1954.

KISSEN, D. M., and LE SHAN, L. L. (eds.), *Psychosomatic Aspects of Neoplastic Disease.* London, Pitman Medical Publishing Company, Ltd., 1964.

KOWAL, S. J., "Emotions as a Cause of Cancer: 18th and 19th Century Contributions." *Psychoanalytic Review,* Vol. 42, 217-227, 1955.

LA BARBA, R. C., "Experimental Factors in Cancer: A Review of Research with Animals." *Psychosomatic Medicine,* Vol, 32, 259-275.

LE SHAN, L. "Personality States as Factors in the Development of Malignant Disease: A Critical Review." *Journal of the National Cancer Institute,* Vol. 22, 1-18, 1959.

———, "Some Methodological Problems in the Study of the Psychosomatic Aspects of Cancer." *Journal of General Psychology,* Vol. 63, 309-317, 1960.

———, and WORTHINGTON, R. E., "Personality as a Factor in the Pathogenesis of Cancer: A Review of the Literature." *British Journal of Medical Psychology,* Vol. 29, 49-56, 1956.

MEERLOO, J., "Psychological Implications of Malignant Growth: Survey of Hypotheses." *British Journal of Medical Psychology,* Vol. 27, 210-215, 1954.

Research on Specific Aspects of the Field

ANDERVONT, H. B., "Influence of Environment on Mammary Cancer in Mice." *Journal of the National Cancer Institute*, Vol. 4, 579-581, 1944.

BACON, C. L., RENNECKER, R., and CUTLER, M. A., "A Psychosomatic Survey of Cancer of the Breast." *Psychosomatic Medicine*, Vol. 14, 453-460, 1952.

BAHNSON, C. B., *Basic Epistemological Problems Regarding Psychosomatic Processes*. Paper Presented at the First International Congress on Higher Nervous Activity, Milan, 1968.

EVANS, E. A. *A Psychological Study of Cancer*. New York, Dodd-Mead and Co., 1926.

FISHER, S., and CLEVELAND, S. E., "Relationship of Body Image to Site of Cancer." *Psychosomatic Medicine*, Vol. 18, 304-309, 1956.

FOQUE, E., "Le Problem de Cancer dans ses Aspects Psychiques." *Gazette Hôpital*, Paris, Vol. 104, 827-833, 1931.

GREENE, W. A., "Psychological Factors and Reticuloendothelial Diseases, 1." *Psychosomatic Medicine*, Vol. 16, 220-230, 1954.

————, YOUNG, L., and SWISHER, S. N., "Psychological Factors and Reticuloendothelial Disease, 2." *Psychosomatic Medicine*, Vol. 18, 284-303, 1956.

————, and MILLER, G., "Psychological Factors and Reticuloendothelial Disease, 4." *Psychosomatic Medicine*, Vol. 20, 122-144, 1958.

KISSEN, D. M., "Personality Factors in Males Conducive

to Lung Cancer," *British Journal of Medical Psychology,* Vol. 36, p. 27, 1963.

———, "Psychosocial Factors, Personality and Lung Cancer in Men Aged 55-64." *British Journal of Medical Psychology,* Vol. 40, p. 29, 1967.

———, and EYSENCK, H. G., "Personality in Male Lung Cancer Patients." *Journal of Psychosomatic Research,* Vol. 6, p. 123, 1962.

———, "Relationship Between Lung Cancer, Cigarette Smoking, Inhalation, and Personality and Psychological Factors." *British Journal of Medical Psychology,* Vol. 37, 344-351, 1964.

KLOPFER, B., "Psychological Factors in Human Cancer." *Journal of Projective Techniques,* Vol. 21, 331-340, 1957.

LE SHAN, L. and WORTHINGTON, R. E., "Some Psychologic Correlates of Neoplastic Disease: Preliminary Report." *Journal of Clinical and Experimental Psychopathology,* Vol. 16, 281-288, 1955.

———, "Loss of Cathexes as a Common Psychodynamic Characteristic of Cancer Patients." *Psychological Reports,* Vol. 2, 183-193, 1956.

———, "Some Recurrent Life History Patterns Observed in Patients with Malignant Disease." *Journal of Nervous and Mental Disease,* Vol. 124, 460-465, 1956.

———, "A Psychosomatic Hypothesis Concerning the Etiology of Hodgkin's Disease." *Psychological Reports,* Vol. 3, 565-575, 1957.

———, and GASSMAN, M. "Some Observations on Psychotherapy with Patients with Neoplastic Disease."

American Journal of Psychotherapy, Vol. 12, 723-734, 1958.

————, MARVIN, S., and LYERLY, O., "Some Evidence of a Relationship Between Hodgkin's Disease and Intelligence." *American Medical Association Archives of General Psychiatry,* Vol. 1, 447-449, 1959.

————, and REZNIKOFF, M., "A Psychological Factor Apparently Associated with Neoplastic Disease." *Journal of Abnormal and Social Psychology,* Vol. 60, 439-440, 1960.

————, "A Basic Psychological Orientation Apparently Associated with Neoplastic Disease." *Psychiatric Quarterly,* April 1961, 1-17.

————, and LESHAN, E., "Psychotherapy and the Patient with a Limited Life Span." *Psychiatry,* Vol. 24, 318-323, 1961.

MILLER, F. R., and JONES, H. W., "The Possibility of Precipitating the Leukemic State by Emotional Factors." *Blood,* Vol. 8, 880-884, 1948.

PELLER, S. *Cancer in Man.* New York, International University Press, 1962.

REZNIKOFF, M., "Psychological Factors in Breast Cancer." *Psychosomatic Medicine,* Vol. 18, p. 2, 1955.

————, and MARTIN, P. E., "The Influence of Stress on Mammary Cancer in Mice." *Journal of Psychosomatic Research,* Vol. 2, 56-60, 1957.

SIMONTON, J. C., and SIMONTON, S., "Belief Systems and Management of the Emotional Aspects of Malignancy." *Journal of Transpersonal Psychology,* Vol. 7, 29-47, 1975.

SNOW, H. *Clinical Notes on Cancer.* London, J. and A. Churchill, 1883.

THOMAS, C. B., and DUSZYNSKI, D. R., "Closeness to Parents and the Family Constellation in a Prospective Study of Five Disease States: Suicide, Mental Illness, Malignant Tumor, Hypertension, and Coronary Heart Disease." *The John Hopkins Medical Journal,* Vol. 134, 251-270, 1974.

WALSHE, W. A. *The Nature and Treatment of Cancer.* London, Taylor and Walton, 1846.

WEST, P. M., BLUMBERG, E. M., and ELLIS, F., "An Observed Correlation Between Psychological Factors and Growth Rate of Cancer in Man." *Cancer Research,* Vol. 12, 306-307, 1952.

Those professionals who wish to keep up with the development of this field should write to:

Dr. H. J. F. Baltrush
Chairman
European Working Group for Psychosomatic
Cancer Research (EUPSYCA)
Bergstrasse 10
D-2900 Oldenburg
Federal Republic of Germany